Psychological Factors Affecting Medical Conditions

Advances in Psychosomatic Medicine

Vol. 28

Series Editor

T.N. Wise, Falls Church, Va.

Editors

G.A. Fava, Bologna
I. Fukunishi, Tokyo
M.B. Rosenthal, Cleveland, Ohio

Psychological Factors Affecting Medical Conditions

A New Classification for DSM-V

Volume Editors

P. Porcelli, Castellana Grotte
N. Sonino, Padova

3 figures and 22 tables, 2007

KARGER

Basel · Freiburg · Paris · London · New York ·
Bangalore · Bangkok · Singapore · Tokyo · Sydney

Advances in Psychosomatic Medicine

Founded 1960 by
F. Deutsch (Cambridge, Mass.)
A. Jores (Hamburg)
B. Stockvis (Leiden)

Continued 1972–1982 by
F. Reichsman (Brooklyn, N.Y.)

Library of Congress Cataloging-in-Publication Data

Psychological factors affecting medical conditions : a new classification
for DSM-V / volume editors, P. Porcelli, N. Sonino.
p. ; cm. – (Advances in psychosomatic medicine, ISSN 0065-3268 ; v.
28)
Includes bibliographical references and indexes.
ISBN-13: 978-3-8055-8331-2 (hard cover : alk. paper)
1. Medicine, Psychosomatic–Research–Methodology. 2.
Sick–Psychology–Classification. 3. Diseases–Social
aspects–Classification. 4. Diagnostic and statistical manual of mental
disorders. I. Porcelli, P. (Piero) II. Sonino, N. (Nicoletta) III.
Diagnostic and statistical manual of mental disorders. IV. Series.
[DNLM: 1. Psychophysiologic Disorders–classification. 2.
Psychophysiologic Disorders–diagnosis. 3. Disease–psychology. 4.
Psychosomatic Medicine–methods. 5. Research. W1 AD81 v.28 2007 / WM 90
P97147 2007]
RC52.P82 2007
616.08–dc22

2007025224

Bibliographic Indices. This publication is listed in bibliographic services, including Current Contents® and Index Medicus.

www.karger.com
Printed in Switzerland on acid-free and non-aging paper (ISO 9706) by Reinhardt Druck, Basel
ISSN 0065–3268
ISBN 978–3–8055–8331–2

Contents

Preface

The primary goals of diagnosis are to provide clinicians with a meaningful framework that recognizes the underlying clinical condition beyond the symptom presentation, to facilitate communication among clinicians, and to enhance decision making to improve the patient's health status. In any field of medicine and clinical psychology, including psychosomatic medicine, the diagnostic process can be considered as much effective as it gets closer to the top achievement levels of these 3 interrelated purposes. However, a wide array of medical symptoms cannot be explained by the biomedical model and confined to the current branches of internal medicine. In turn, several health-related problems, strongly affecting daily functioning and influencing symptom presentation, cannot be fully recognized without the more comprehensive, multifactorial perspective provided by the biopsychosocial model of health and illness. In this perspective, any illness is viewed as the common final pathway resulting from interacting systems at the cellular, tissue, organismic, interpersonal, and environmental levels, so that each of these factors has a relative weight in facilitating, sustaining, or modifying the course of diseases, varying from illness to illness, from one individual to another, and even between two different episodes of the same illness in the same individual. The relationships between physical illness and psychological factors are subsumed in two chapters of the DSM-IV. One, Somatoform Disorders, is included in the main diagnostic axis I and is based on the assumptions that somatic symptoms are likely to mimic 'real' symptoms of medical disease while not showing any evidence of it and are not secondary to another psychiatric disorder. This view pertains to the concept of the excessive distance between the physical problem (inexistent or not being a plausible cause for actual symptoms) and the patient's perception, thoughts, and behavior. The second chapter is the rubric of Psychological Factors Affecting Medical Condition (PFAMC) that requires the presence of a general medical condition and of psychological factors that adversely affect the course or treatment of the condition, or that increase physical or emotional risk for the patient. PFAMC are placed in the residual section of 'other conditions that may be a focus of clinical attention' and therefore are too vague, lack specific criteria, and are not uscful and not used in clinical practice. Somatoform disorders have attracted considerable criticism since their introduction in the DSM-III and the need for considerable changes in preparing the 5th edition of the DSM has been highlighted. Somatoform disorders have been criticized because they have been formulated by dichotomous thinking; they include criteria that are too restrictive (e.g. somatization disorder) or too vague (e.g. undifferentiated somatoform disorders); they tend to overpsychologize somatic symptoms (when axis I disorders are present) or to underestimate somatization symptoms (when medical diagnoses are established); they underestimate the prevalence of somatization because they are limited to the more severe clinical forms; they underrecognize the dimensional nature of somatization along a continuum spectrum of degrees (severity, impairment, chronicity, comorbidity, health care utilization); they lack appropriate consideration of subsyndromal symptoms, personality and behavioral factors, and they include syndromes that are not used by physicians for the same illness (such as fibromyalgia and undifferentiated somatoform disorder or functional abdominal pain and pain disorder), thereby producing ineffective communication. Both Somatoform Disorders and PFAMC miss the primary goals of the diagnostic process. The debate is still ongoing, several papers and editorials have been published recently, and some proposals for DSM-V have been advanced. They range from softer (e.g. clustering of the many somatoform disorders in few categories identified by some specifiers) to harder alternatives (e.g. abolition of the rubric of somatoform disorders).

On the basis of a growing body of research, this volume deals with research data and clinical views to formulate a new proposal for the DSM-V, introducing the Diagnostic Criteria for Psychosomatic Research (DCPR) in the chapter of PFAMC. The DCPR syndromes were developed about 10 years ago by an international group of investigators and are based on the recognition that a wide body of evidence that has accumulated in psychosomatic medicine relating to concepts of quality of life, stressful life events, somatization, and personality disorders has not resulted in operational tools whereby different psychosocial aspects of medical diseases can be characterized. The DCPR approach focuses on psychological characteristics of patients presenting symptoms across different medical disorders.

The first chapter by Fabbri and colleagues explains the rationale for the introduction of the DCPR in the DSM-V and emphasizes their usefulness assessing for psychological and behavioral problems affecting the onset, the course, and the treatment of patients in the different medical settings. In the second chapter, Sonino and colleagues examine the psychological factors affecting several endocrine disorders (Cushing's syndrome, Graves' disease, Addison's disease, primary aldosteronism, thyroid dysfunctions, hyperprolactinemia, and hyperparathyroidism). Particular attention is paid by the authors to the association between DCPR clusters and the construct of allostatic load, conceived as the chronic exposure to fluctuating or heightened neuroendocrine response resulting from repeated or chronic environmental challenge. Porcelli and Todarello's chapter focuses on patients with functional gastrointestinal disorders in whom the most prevalent DCPR syndromes (alexithymia, persistent somatization, secondary functional somatic symptoms, and demoralization) are consistent with the psychosocial correlates outlined in the literature as health care seeking behavior and somatosensory amplification. In the following chapter, Grassi and coworkers underscore that DSM criteria are particularly problematic in oncology because of the need to adapt them to the cancer-related life conditions, while psychological problems identified by the DCPR as health anxiety, demoralization, and alexithymia are associated with several cancer-related physical symptoms, poor well-being and quality of life, and high health concerns. The psychological factors affecting cardiovascular disorders are reviewed by Rafanelli's group. In this chapter, the role of 'classic' (stressful life events, depression, anxiety, anger, and hostility) and DCPR-related (demoralization, health anxiety, irritable mood, type A behavior, and denial) psychological factors are discussed in relation to coronary heart disease, essential hypertension, congestive heart failure, heart transplantation, coronary artery bypass grafting, and cardiac rehabilitation. In the subsequent chapter, Picardi and Pasquini review the psychological factors (demoralization, type A behavior, secondary somatic symptoms, irritable mood, and health anxiety) that influence dermatological conditions such as alopecia aerata, atopic dermatitis, psoriasis, and vitiligo. The skin is a sensory organ involved in socialization processes, which is responsive to various emotional stimuli, and affects an individual's body image and self-esteem. The last two chapters are concerned with two areas closer to psychiatry. Bellomo's group highlights findings on psychological factors in the setting of consultation-liaison psychiatry and Fassino and colleagues discuss issues of patients with eating disorders. Both conditions have important biological and psychiatric determinants involved in the presentation and the treatment of symptoms and require a multidisciplinary approach in order to provide highly integrated management. Finally, two appendices report the complete list of criteria for the 12 DCPR categories and the structured interview for their assessment.

The goal of this volume is to provide the best tools in diagnosing psychosocial correlates of medical disorders. The distinct DCPR categories are consistent with concepts expressed by a large body of research and outstanding authors in psychosomatic medicine and are therefore suggested as specifiers of 'psychological factors affecting medical conditions' in the future DSM-V. The aim of the DCPR is to translate psychological characteristics observed in various medical settings into operational criteria, which may entail clinical value, and may be studied across disorders, regardless of their supposed functional or organic nature. The review papers included in the present volume strongly support the use of the DCPR in medical settings and hopefully will generate interest for a more effective clinical practice.

Piero Porcelli, PhD
Nicoletta Sonino, MD

Porcelli P, Sonino N (eds): Psychological Factors Affecting Medical Conditions. A New Classification for DSM-V. Adv Psychosom Med. Basel, Karger, 2007, vol 28, pp 1–20

Development of a New Assessment Strategy in Psychosomatic Medicine: The Diagnostic Criteria for Psychosomatic Research

Stefania Fabbri[a,b], *Giovanni A. Fava*[a,c], *Laura Sirri*[a], *Thomas N. Wise*[d]

[a]Department of Psychology, University of Bologna, Bologna, Italy; [b]Department of Psychiatry and Neurobehavioral Sciences, University of Virginia, Charlottesville, Va., [c]Department of Psychiatry, State University of New York at Buffalo, Buffalo, N.Y., [d]Department of Psychiatry and Behavioral Sciences, Johns Hopkins University, Baltimore, Md., USA

Abstract

The Diagnostic Criteria for Psychosomatic Research (DCPR) are a diagnostic and conceptual framework that was proposed a decade ago by an international group of investigators. The DCPR's rationale was to translate psychosocial variables that derived from psychosomatic research into operational tools whereby individual patients could be identified. A set of 12 syndromes was developed: health anxiety, thanatophobia, disease phobia, illness denial, persistent somatization, conversion symptoms, functional somatic symptoms secondary to a psychiatric disorder, anniversary reaction, demoralization, irritable mood, type A behavior, and alexithymia. These criteria were meant to be used in a multiaxial approach. The aim of this work is to survey the research evidence which has accumulated on the DCPR, to provide specification for their development and validation and to examine the specific DCPR clusters. Their implications for classification purposes (DSM-V) are also discussed.

The last decade has witnessed an increased interest in the assessment of those psychological factors that may modulate the vulnerability to or the course, prognosis and rehabilitation of physical diseases.

The chapter on somatoform disorders, which was introduced in the DSM-III [1] and retained in its subsequent editions, has become a key tool for performing such assessment. From the very beginning, the classification of somatoform disorders has attracted considerable criticism for its failure to adequately cover the clinical phenomena of somatization [1–8], defined by Lipowski [4] as the tendency to experience and communicate psychological distress in the form of physical symptoms and to seek medical help for them. Part of the problem has been the process for development of the somatoform disorders within the DSM iterations. The committee that developed the criteria also was charged with establishing criteria for impulse and dissociative disorders. Furthermore, the committee did not include the many international investigators whose careers have focused upon such somatoform issues. It is thus not surprising that the current taxonomy is limited from both an evidence-based perspective as well as from a clinical vantage point.

Recently, Mayou et al. [5] suggested that the DSM-V abolished the diagnostic category of somatoform disorders and redistributed some of its current diagnoses into other groupings. Hypochondriasis should be renamed as 'health anxiety disorder' and placed together with body-dysmorphic disorder within anxiety disturbances. Somatization disorder would be defined by a combination of personality disorder (axis II) with mood or anxiety disorders (axis I). Somatic symptoms and syndromes and pain disorder could be classified on axis III for reporting current general medical conditions. Dissociative and conversion symptoms would stay on their own [5].

Hiller and Rief [9] and Noyes et al. [10] acknowledged that the classification of somatoform disorders lacks support in many areas and requires substantial modifications. However, they suggested that the diagnoses of hypochondriasis and somatization disorders have traditionally been recognized, are clinically distinct forms of somatic distress, and entail prognostic and therapeutic implications [9, 10].

Mayou et al. [5] advocated a greater use of 'psychological factors affecting medical condition' on axis I. However they did not provide further indications which may help the clinician in implementing this shift. The essential features of the diagnosis are the presence of a general medical condition and of psychological factors adversely affecting its course and treatment or constituting health risks and stress-related physiological responses. Examples are provided by major depression in the setting of myocardial infarction, symptoms of anxiety and depression affecting the course and the severity of irritable bowel syndrome, type A personality in coronary artery disease, unsafe lifestyle and stressful life situations precipitating pain.

It thus appears that the focus of assessment of current strategies based on DSM is too narrow and/or misplaced and is not in line with the spectrum of manifestations of psychological distress and illness behavior in the medical setting which have resulted from the use of dimensional tools (particularly self-rating scales).

A diagnostic and conceptual framework was proposed a decade ago by an international group of investigators [11]. The rationale of these Diagnostic

Criteria for Psychosomatic Research (DCPR) was to translate psychosocial variables that were derived from psychosomatic research into operational tools whereby individual patients could be identified. A set of 12 diagnostic criteria was developed. These criteria were meant to be used in a multiaxial approach.

Some of the DCPR clusters were based on Pilowsky's concept of abnormal illness behavior, characterized as the persistence of a maladaptive mode of perceiving, experiencing, evaluating, and responding to one's health status, despite the fact that a doctor has provided a lucid and accurate appraisal of the situation and management to be followed, if any, with opportunities for discussion, negotiation, and clarification, based on adequate assessment of all relevant biological, psychological, social and cultural factors [12]. Health anxiety, hypochondriasis and disease phobia pertain to the illness-affirming expressions, whereas illness denial to the illness denying modalities. All types of DCPR may occur in conjunction with psychiatric disorders listed in the DSM-IV such as major depressive episodes or panic disorder, or medical disorders, regardless of the functional/organic dichotomy.

The aim of this work was to survey the research evidence which has accumulated on the DCPR.

We will first provide specification for the DCPR development and validation and then examine the specific clusters.

The Diagnostic Criteria for Psychosomatic Research

The DCPR consist of a set of 12 'psychosomatic syndromes', developed with the aim to translate psychosocial variables of prognostic and therapeutic value in the course of physical conditions into categorical criteria (see appendix 1). The 12 clusters are concerned with alexithymia, type A behavior, disease phobia, thanatophobia, health anxiety, illness denial, functional somatic symptoms secondary to psychiatric disorders, persistent somatization, conversion symptoms, anniversary reactions, irritable mood and demoralization. Despite their clinical importance, these areas have been neglected by traditional psychiatric nosography, mainly because of their subsyndromic nature.

The specific criteria included in each of the DCPR clusters represent the most relevant features of the related syndrome, as evidenced by reviewing pertaining psychosomatic literature.

Since their development, several studies found the DCPR more suitable than DSM-IV and ICD-10 [13] criteria in identifying psychological distress and impaired quality of life both in patients with medical, functional or psychiatric disorders and in the general population [14–30].

A structured interview [26] was developed to assess the presence of the 12 syndromes. It showed excellent interrater reliability (with κ-values ranging from 0.69 to 0.97) [15], with good correlations with dimensional instruments for the assessment of psychosocial distress, such as the Toronto Alexithymia Scale [14, 31], the Psychosocial Index [29] and the General Health Questionnaire [22]. Both quantitative and qualitative differences emerged between the DCPR and DSM-IV systems. In fact, the psychosomatic syndromes were not only more prevalent (about double) than the psychiatric disorders, but they frequently led to the identification of psychosocial distress in the absence of a DSM-IV diagnosis. Furthermore, some evidence suggested that DCPR and DSM-IV categories are not linked by a hierarchical relationship. This was particularly evident in the case of demoralization and major depression: not all patients with depression also present with demoralization and vice versa. Finally, DCPR diagnoses significantly predicted the treatment outcome of patients with functional gastrointestinal disorders (FGID) [25].

The DCPR criteria dealing with type A behavior, irritable mood and demoralization syndromes require the presence of a specific relationship between psychological symptoms and the precipitation or exacerbation of a medical condition, mainly through the elicitation of stress-related physiologic responses. Traditional psychometric tools, both categorical and dimensional, are limited to subjective expressions (cognitive, affective and behavioral), yet they do not add anything to the understanding on how those psychological clusters modulate physical status. For example, it has been proposed that the mixed results about the predictive role of type A behavior in cardiovascular vulnerability could depend on the instruments adopted for its identification [32]. DCPR diagnoses may represent an attempt to overcome this problem, putting the relationship with physiological alterations as key identification criteria.

Health Anxiety

Pilowsky's concept [12] of abnormal illness behavior, Kellner's work derived from the use of the Illness Attitude Scale (IAS) [33–35] and more recent literature [36] suggest that the differential diagnosis between hypochondriasis, disease phobia, thanatophobia and health anxiety is worthy of clinical attention and may entail prognostic and therapeutic implications.

Health anxiety may encompass nonspecific dimensions of abnormal illness behavior, such as generic worries about illness, concerns about pain and bodily preoccupations (accompanied by the tendency to amplify somatic sensations). In the case of health anxiety, worries and fears about health readily respond to appropriate reassurance, characteristic element that differentiates health anxiety from hypochondrias. These forms of health anxiety may be short-lived unlike hypochondriasis, disease phobia and thanatophobia that tend to persist over time [37].

Grassi et al. [17] reported that 55 out of 159 oncology patients (37.7%) met the criteria for health anxiety, Porcelli et al. [24] reported that health anxiety was present in 11.6% of patients suffering from FGID and Grandi et al. [16] found that 7.7% of patients that underwent a heart transplant presented with health anxiety. Porcelli et al. [25] in a later study, aimed to identify predictors of treatment outcome in patients undergoing treatment for FGID found that the DCPR category of health anxiety was significantly more prevalent in improved (21.5%) than unimproved (2.5%) patients. Health anxiety was also found to be a significant independent predictor of improvement.

Thanatophobia

In 1928, Ryle [38] described this syndrome as the sense of dying (angor animi). About 20 years later, he provided the following lucid, autobiographical description of the symptoms:

> 'It had never occurred to me that I should have an actual opportunity of observing the symptoms in my own person until the autumn of 1942, when I developed angina pectoris. . . My first manifestation (. . .) was a sudden and intense attack of the sense of dying. I had just climbed the stairs of the refectory at the medical school at Guy's and sat down to lunch when it swept upon me. I remember thinking to myself in the very words employed over the radio by a gallant fighter pilot as he fell to his death, 'This is it' and I could not doubt that I was about to die. The sensation then as afterwards passed in a few seconds. On several subsequent occasions I was almost as convinced that the end had come. Thereafter I must have experienced the symptoms, in varying degree, probably on 200 or more occasions within a period of 5 or 6 years, and I have long since come to accept it philosophically.'

Kellner [33] associated the conviction of dying soon (although for no objective reason) with the fear of news which reminds of death, such as funerals of obituary notices. Thanatophobia may occur in the setting of hypochondriasis [35], panic disorder [39], and disease phobia [40]. In the latter condition, the phobic quality of these fears may result in panic attacks. Morselli [41] also differentiates that fear of dying that manifests itself in isolated attacks of intense quality in phobic patients from the more chronic worry of melancholic patients. Mayer-Gross et al. [42] remark the association between the idea and fear of death and obsessive illness. However, thanatophobia may occur also in the absence of other psychological symptoms. Its prevalence in medical patients deserves attention.

More recent studies that investigated the prevalence of thanatophobia in the medical setting have found that criteria for thanatophobia were met by 8.2% of oncology patients [17], 6.9% of transplanted patients [16], 4.9% of subjects in cardiac rehabilitation [26], and 1.6% of patients with FGID [24].

Disease Phobia

Bianchi [43] has defined disease phobia (nosophobia) as 'a persistent, unfounded fear of suffering from a disease, with some doubt remaining despite examination and reassurance'. Ryle [44] included in disease phobia the fear of inheriting or acquiring a disease and attributed a causal role to medical articles published in lay press.

Disease phobia is often secondary to hypochondriasis, yet it may also be observed in the absence of other psychiatric disorders deserving a proper nosological status and specific therapeutic implications [45, 46]. Despite this, up to the development of DCPR, disease phobia has been neglected by psychiatric nosography and very few dimensional tools allow its quantitative assessment. One of the nine IAS was specifically focused on disease phobia [34] and later inspired the homonymous DCPR cluster. A scale for disease phobia also emerged from the factorial analysis of the Whiteley Index [47] and, together with the IAS, proved to be very valid and sensitive in differentiating hypochondriasis from somatization [9].

Differential diagnosis between hypochondriacal beliefs and disease phobia is worthy of clinical attention and may entail prognostic and therapeutic implications.

Fava and Grandi [36] underlined two main clinical features of disease phobia. The first one is the specificity and longitudinal stability of the symptoms (e.g. patients who fear to have cancer are unlikely to transfer their fear to another disease, AIDS for example). In hypochondriacal patients, on the contrary, a switch in the object of fear is likely to occur over time. The second characteristic of disease phobia is the phobic quality of the fears [40] that tend to manifest themselves in attacks rather than in constant, chronic worries like in hypochondriasis. Those two main phenomenological differences between hypochondriasis and disease phobia lead to different therapeutic approaches. Warwick and Marks [48] successfully used exposure to illness cues and prevention of reassurance with 17 subjects suffering from disease phobia. The phobic quality of the fear, typical of disease phobia, often leads to avoidance that can be faced with in vivo exposure. In contrast, the constant fear of diseases characteristic of hypochondriacal patients often leads to doctor shopping behaviors that may not respond to exposure. In this sense, the relationship of disease phobia to hypochondriasis is similar to the one of panic disorder to generalized anxiety [36]. Further, disease phobia was found to respond to imipramine, unlike hypochondriasis [49].

Using the DCPR, disease phobia has a nonmarginal prevalence in clinical populations, since this syndrome was identified in a percentage of subjects varying from 2.2% in dermatological patients [23] to 19% in consultation-liaison psychiatry patients [15].

Illness Denial

The concept of denial derived from psychoanalytic theory indicating an ego-defense mechanism against unpleasant feelings [50]. Later, denial was included among the emotion-focused coping strategies engaged by people when a stressful situation has to be faced [51].

In the conceptual framework of abnormal illness behavior [12], illness denial represents a psychological response to one's own illness and covers several phenomenological phenomena ranging from an unrealistic optimism to the complete denial of disease. According to the broad spectrum of illness-related features that can be denied, distorted or minimized, many components of illness denial have been identified [52]. For instance, patients can deny urgency, seriousness, affect, personal relevance, responsibility, long-term prognosis (including the possibility of death), implications of the diagnosis, the need of therapy [52, 53].

Denial of physical illness has been described in a variety of clinical settings, especially in patients with cancer, diabetes, renal, cardiovascular and neurological disorders [15, 52, 54–56]. Much has been debated about the adaptive/maladaptive role of illness denial [51, 52]. In the early stage of life-threatening diseases, after diagnosis, and in the terminal phase, a certain degree of denial alleviates psychological distress and in women with nonmetastatic breast cancer may be associated with a longer survival [55].

Denial is termed as maladaptive when it prevents the adoption of healthy behaviors and results in a delay in seeking medical care and nonadherence to therapies or lifestyle modification programs [51]. In these cases, denial may worsen the course of disease, as was found to occur in diabetic patients where it was associated with hematic markers of poor metabolic control [54]. Nonacceptance of illness may be displayed by counterphobic behavior; this is the case of the hemophilic patient who engages in risky behaviors. In healthy subjects, illness denial may represent a risk factor for unsafe health habits, as found for HIV/AIDS-related denial [57].

Despite its clinical relevance, maladaptive illness denial has been neglected by psychiatric classifications [13, 58]. Some authors proposed the inclusion of denial in the DSM-IV as a subtype of adjustment disorder [59–61], whilst distinctive criteria for the recognition of denial in physical illness have been provided by the DCPR [11]. DCPR criteria for illness denial identified this phenomenon in several clinical contexts, with a prevalence ranging from 2% in dermatological inpatients [22] to 29% in consultation-liaison psychiatry patients [15].

Persistent Somatization

Somatization is a widespread clinical phenomenon which cuts across diagnostic categories, both of psychiatric and medical type.

Kellner [3] summarized some characteristics of patients suffering from various functional medical disorders, such as nonulcer dyspepsia, urethral syndrome and irritable bowel syndrome. He also suggested that it may be advantageous to conceptualize a somatizing patient as someone in whom psychophysiological symptoms have clustered.

The DCPR category of persistent somatization attempts to overcome some conceptual flaws of the DSM-IV diagnosis of somatization disorder, which appears to be rarely used and of limited utility in clinical settings, mostly because of its very restrictive criteria [62].

Recently, various studies in different medical settings have used DCPR in order to assess the frequency and characteristics of persistent somatization. The prevalence of the syndrome ranged from 1.5% in heart-transplanted patients [16] to 21% in endocrine patients [29]. In a sample of 190 subjects suffering from FGID [24], the percentage of patients meeting the criteria for persistent somatization goes up even higher reaching as much as 38%. In this study, in more than 2 out of 3 cases, persistent somatization was not associated with DSM somatoform disorders and thus somatization phenomena that would have otherwise been missed could be detected. This phenomenon can be explained by the fact that, despite the fact that the criteria for persistent somatization are more selective than those used to define undifferentiated somatoform disorder, the former could be diagnosed also in the presence of a comorbid psychiatric condition. Interestingly, DCPR persistent somatization seldom occurred in a community sample [20].

According to evidence, cognitive-behavioral strategies represent the preferable psychological treatment for somatization. In a review [63] of 31 controlled studies, cognitive-behavioral therapy for somatization had a superior result to control conditions in 71% of the studies.

Conversion Symptoms

Symptoms or deficits affecting voluntary motor or sensory function that are not explained by organic causes are often labeled as 'conversion symptoms'.

The differentiation between somatization disorder and conversion according to DSM-IV is mainly based on the number of symptoms instead of more precise clinical features. In their review article, Stone et al. [64] highlighted that a misdiagnosis of conversion symptoms was reported in early studies but this rate reached a level of only 4% in studies after 1970. The authors explain this decline '. . . as probably due to improvements in study quality rather than improved diagnostic accuracy. . .', pointing out how the difficulties in making a diagnosis of conversion disorder are still prevalent.

According to the DSM-IV classification, the diagnosis of a conversion disorder is frequently made by exclusion of another somatoform disorder or a medical condition. Yet, Engel [65] provided a set of more stringent criteria, which lead to a definition of conversion symptoms.

One of Engel's criteria is concerned with ambivalence in symptom reporting (e.g. the patient appears relaxed or unconcerned as he describes distressing symptoms). This definition only partially overlaps with the DSM 'la belle indifférence', which has not been found to be a discriminatory symptom of conversion [66]. Engel's criteria were incorporated in the DCPR diagnostic criteria for conversion symptoms.

The identification of conversion phenomena is made more difficult by the observation that symptoms ascribed to a conversion process may frequently represent a prodromal phase of a medical, mainly neurological, disorder [67].

Porcelli et al. [24] found that 5% of subjects suffering form FGID present with DCPR conversion symptoms and Ottolini et al. [21], in a population of subjects on their first episode of myocardial infarction, found conversion symptoms in 7% of the patients. This confirms previous findings on the occurrence of conversion symptoms also in the setting of life-threatening medical illness [67].

The treatment of conversion symptoms should be multifaced, combining psychopharmacotherapy and psychotherapy [68–71].

Functional Somatic Symptoms Secondary to a Psychiatric Disorder

Psychosomatic research in the field of functional symptoms had suggested a high percentage of psychiatric comorbidity [2], and a primary-secondary distinction had been found to be feasible [72]. This diagnosis allows to establish a hierarchical relationship between psychiatric morbidity and the onset of functional medical disorders, which would otherwise be subsumed under the not particularly clinically meaningful rubric of comorbidity. This hierarchical rule was found to have clinical and predictive value [73].

In the study of Porcelli et al. [24], 29.9% of patients with FGID were found to have Functional Somatic Symptoms Secondary to a Psychiatric Disorder. Interestingly, in more than half of the cases of mood and anxiety disorders, FGID were not judged to be secondary to a psychiatric disorder.

Anniversary Reaction

The relationship between anniversaries and the onset or exacerbation of illness has been of long-standing clinical interest, particularly as to how anniversaries reactivate old repressed and unresolved conflicts [74]. Hilgard [75] observed that symptoms may be precipitated in a parent when the parent's child reaches the age at which the parent had experienced a traumatic episode in childhood. In a subsequent report, Hilgard and Newman [76] extended the precipitating trigger situation to include the age of the adult patient as it coincides with the age of the parent who died during the patient's childhood. Anniversaries do not need to be tied to age, but may be related to other periodicities. The concept of nemesis [77] is closely related to anniversary reactions. The patient believes he or she is destined to repeat in his or her life the pattern of a significant other person's life which ended in tragedy or catastrophe. Engel [74] outlined the links between anniversaries and the giving up-given up complex.

The DCPR criteria for anniversary reaction may be a special form of conversion as well as other types of somatization. Grandi et al. [16] found that 0.7% of patients undergoing heart transplantation presented with anniversary reaction and Porcelli et al. [24] found a similar figure (0.5%) of anniversary reaction in patients with FGID.

Demoralization

According to Frank [78], demoralization represents the common reason why subjects seek psychotherapeutic treatment and results from the consciousness of being unable to cope with a pressing problem, or of having failed one's own expectations or those of others [79].

Several definitions of demoralization have been proposed, ranging from 'a normal response to adversity' [80] and 'a non-specific psychological distress' [81] to a specific syndrome resulting from the convergence of distress and subjective incompetence [82].

Schmale and Engel [83] identified a psychological state, the so-called 'giving up-given up syndrome' that clearly describes the distinctive features of demoralization and is characterized by feelings of helplessness, hopelessness, subjective incompetence and loss of mastery and control. This syndrome was found to frequently occur before the onset of medical disorders and can be exacerbated or triggered by a physical illness, especially if life-threatening or disabling, or by painful and prolonged treatments, such as chemotherapy and mastectomy [80, 83].

Hopelessness, the most relevant feature of demoralization, independently from depression, was associated with suicidal intent and action in both medical and psychiatric patients [84] and seemed to increase the risk and worsen the prognosis of cardiovascular diseases and cancer [84–86].

Despite its clinical and prognostic relevance, demoralization has not been adequately recognized by traditional psychiatric classifications and a very few dimensional instruments have been specifically developed for its assessment. The most relevant are the Demoralization Scale of the Psychiatric Epidemiology Research Interview [81] and the Beck Hopelessness Scale [87].

The application of the DCPR operational criteria has permitted to document the occurrence of demoralization across different medical settings, substantiating previous findings that used dimensional tools [88, 89]. Demoralization was found to be one of the most frequent psychosomatic syndromes in medically ill patients, with a prevalence of almost 30% [15–18, 22, 24, 29]. In cardiology, it has been identified as a prodromal symptom of cardiac events [21, 27]. Demoralization appeared to be far less frequent among subjects recruited in a community sample [20]. These findings suggested that demoralization and major depression are overlapping but distinct clinical phenomena, not hierarchically linked: patients can be demoralized but not depressed and vice versa.

Some authors have suggested that demoralization in medically ill patients may be reduced by a regular, supportive and emphatic relationship between the patient and the health care providers [80, 84]. Yet, a specific psychotherapeutic intervention, mainly based on cognitive and behavioral techniques, is required when demoralization becomes chronic and severe [84]. Future studies should clarify whether relief from demoralization results in better illness course and outcome.

Irritable Mood

The most clinically relevant features of irritability have been well described by Snaith and Taylor [90] in the following definition: 'a feeling state characterized by reduced control over temper which usually results in irascible verbal or behavioral outbursts, although the mood may be present without observed manifestation. It may be experienced as brief episodes, in particular circumstances, or it may be prolonged and generalized. The experience of irritability is always unpleasant for the individual and overt manifestation lacks the cathartic effect of justified outbursts of anger'.

Several phenomena related to irritable mood have been differentiated: inward and outward irritability, hostility, aggression and anger are similar but distinct phenomena. Irritable mood can represent a mood state independent of other anxious or depressive disorders [90], yet irritability may be secondary to all the major psychiatric disturbances and type A behavior [91–94].

There are different pathways linking irritability and physical illness [91]. Irritability can be induced by physical illness, as frequently observed in endocrine disorders [29, 95] and may represent a psychological response to hospitalization, disability, pain, treatments and diagnostic procedures, as seen in prenatal examination [91]. However, irritability and other related mood states seemed to be involved in the development of medical diseases [96].

Several findings have evidenced a relationship between hostility, in particular its cynical component, and increased risk of cardiovascular diseases, such as hypertension, atherosclerosis, atrial fibrillation, coronary heart disease (CHD), myocardial infarction, especially in younger subjects [85, 96–98].

Unexpressed anger has been addressed as a predisposing factor to cancer [85], chronic pain and functional somatic symptoms [33]. Increased levels of irritability have been observed both in organic [99, 100] and FGID; in particular anger seemed to influence colon activity [101] and trait anger reactivity predicted the severity of FGID [101]. Further, hostility and irritability were found to be significant predictors of unhealthy behaviors, such as smoking and excessive alcohol consumption [96, 102].

In a sample of 609 outpatients recruited from medical settings, DCPR irritable mood was identified in 27% of patients, while major depression was present in 19% of patients. Even though there was considerable overlap between the two diagnoses, 67% of the patients with major depression were not classified as irritable, and 77% of the patients with irritable mood did not satisfy the criteria for major depression [19].

An important line of research is concerned with treatment of irritable mood and whether such treatment entails beneficial effects on the associated medical illness.

Type A Behavior

The term 'type A behavior' was introduced by the two cardiologists Meyer Friedman and Raymond Rosenman in 1959 [103] to indicate a 'specific emotion-action complex' frequently observed in their patients resulting from the encounter of individual predispositions with particular situations perceived as stressful or challenging. This behavioral pattern was hypothesized to be a strong predisposing factor to CHD.

The type A man was described as 'aggressively involved in a chronic, incessant struggle to achieve more and more in less and less time' [104]. The most relevant features of type A behavior encompass excessive involvement in work and activities subjected to deadlines, time urgency, rapid speech and movements, hostility, competitiveness, desire for achievement. Conversely, these features are reduced or relatively absent in the so-called type B subjects, who are described as calm and easygoing [103].

Compared to type B subjects, type As respond to particular laboratory stressors, perceived as challenging and competitive, with an increased sympathetic nervous system activity, resulting in a greater discharge of catecholamines, especially norepinephrine. Type A behavior appeared to be also associated with a greater activity of the hypothalamic-pituitary-adrenocortical axis, as suggested by higher daily average and peak plasma ACTH values in type A than type B [105].

Both large prospective, as the Western Collaborative Group Study [106] and the Framingham Heart Study [107], and retrospective studies confirmed the relationship between type A behavior and increased cardiovascular morbidity and mortality [32]. In 1981, the accumulated evidence led the National

Heart, Lung and Blood Institute to recognize type A behavior as an independent risk factor for coronary artery disease. Afterwards, however, the studies conducted on the predisposing role of type A behavior in CHD found contradictory results and addressed cynical hostility and time urgency as the two components of type A behavior most predictive of cardiovascular risk [32, 108–110].

Several studies assessed type A behavior with self-administered questionnaires, such as the Jenkins Activity Survey [111], yet semi-structured interviews seem to be more reliable for the recognition of the characteristic motor-expressive signs of type A behavior pattern [11, 26, 107]. DCPR allowed to identify type A behavior also in noncardiological settings, such as consultation-liaison psychiatry patients (11%) [15], patients with skin diseases (12%) [22], FGID (8%) [24] and cancer (8%) [17]. Beresnevaité et al. [14] have performed a multimethod investigation of type A behavior, using also DCPR. The DCPR classification showed high levels of agreement with JAS-SF in measuring type A behavior.

Multifaceted psychological treatments aimed at modifying type A behavior-related lifestyle have been proposed and often resulted in a significant reduction of long-term cardiac recurrences [32, 109, 112–115].

Alexithymia

The term alexithymia was introduced by Sifneos [116] to describe the impoverished fantasy life with a resulting utilitarian way of thinking and a characteristic inability to use appropriate words to describe emotions. Research has shown that the inhibition of emotional expression and particularly a life-long tendency to suppress anger have been found to involve an increased risk for a variety of health problems both using alexithymia or similar psychological constructs [117]. It has also been underlined that alexitymia is more common in patients with long-lasting psychosomatic conditions that in other subjects [117].

Using the DCPR interview, the clinician is able to observe and focus on the patient's emotional responses and therefore capture important pieces of information that would otherwise be lost using a self-rating scale (i.e. Toronto Alexithymia Scale) [117]. Nonetheless, the integration of self-rating instruments and observer-rated ones is always advisable.

Porcelli et al. [24] found that alexithymia, as measured by DCPR and other self-rating measures, appears to be particularly frequent (47.4%) in patients with FGID [24, 118], and the authors also found that the overlap rate between alexithymia and psychiatric diagnoses, particularly mood (66.7 %) and somatoform disorders (48.2 %), is extremely high. This finding supports the results of other research in the field [119–123]. In a more recent paper, Porcelli et al. [25] aimed to evaluate the clinical utility of DCPR in predicting treatment outcome of patients with FGID. They found that the proportion of patients diagnosed with alexithymia was significantly higher in the unimproved (82.2%) than in the improved group (23.1%), and the authors also found that alexithymia was an independent predictor of symptom stability.

Introduced in the 1970s as a psychological characteristic of psychosomatic patients, alexithymia is presently conceived as an unspecific personality trait of vulnerability to disorders of affect dysregulation. A possible explanation for Porcelli's findings might be that alexithymic patients may, on one hand experience more severe somatic symptoms (as a consequence of sustained arousal of the physiological component of emotion response systems) and, on the other hand, may also respond poorly to treatment because of their difficulties in processing emotional and somatic stimuli [124, 125].

Grassi et al. [17] found that 26% of oncology patients present with alexithymia. This study also confirmed Porcelli's finding that underlined a persistent overlap between alexithymia and DSM diagnostic categories such as mood (33.3%) and anxiety disorders (33.3%). Grandi et al. [16] reported that 12.4% of patients undergoing heart transplantation presented with alexithymia.

Conclusions

In the early 60s, Kissen [126] suggested the importance of asking who the patients are, within a given illness population, for whom psychosocial variables are of primary significance, instead of asking which psychological factors give rise to which illness.

The developments of psychosomatic medicine in the subsequent 4 decades [127] have supported his view. Psychosomatic investigators have attempted to demonstrate that a certain psychological characteristic (x) is more prevalent in the condition 'a' compared to the condition 'b'. Even when they did find significant differences by reliable statistical and psychometric methods, this did not mean that every patient with 'a' also presented with 'x' and that a patient with 'b' might not present with 'x' features. Not surprisingly, replication attempts have often been disappointing as one would expect from characteristics of modest sensitivity and low specificity in heterogeneous medical entities [11]. The use of DCPR has disclosed, for instance, that not all coronary artery disease patients display type A behavior [16, 26] and, vice versa, that type A behavior is also present in dermatology [22], gastroenterology [24] and cancer [17] patients.

The development of specific criteria for the DSM category of psychological factors affecting physical condition follows Kissen's strategy [126]: to translate psychological characteristics observed in various medical settings into diagnostic criteria, which may entail clinical (prognostic and therapeutic) value, and may be studied across disorders. These criteria would also fulfill Halliday's wish, expressed 60 years ago [128] of acquiring phenomenological aids that may allow identification of psychosomatic distress across different somatic disorders (whether of functional or organic nature). By using these categories, in the field of functional medical disorders, psychosomatic specialists may bring together a large number of seemingly unrelated disorders whose names have been scattered so far under the headings of the various anatomical systems [128] and pave the ground for multidisciplinary work in clinical medicine [129].

We have proposed to designate Psychological Factors Affecting Medical Conditions as a new section of DSM that consists of the six most frequent DCPR syndromes that have been shown to affect medical conditions [130]. We propose expanding this category with reliable qualifiers to better describe the elements of the psychological factors. The clinical specifiers consist of one DSM-IV somatoform diagnosis (hypochondriasis) and six syndromes which derive from DCPR and the concept of abnormal illness behavior. These syndromes should become the focus of assessment of psychological distress and illness behavior in the setting of medical disease. DCPR were in fact found to be more suitable than DSM-IV criteria in identifying distress and impaired quality of life. These syndromes should be used in conjunction with all other axis I and II diagnoses and would eliminate the need for diagnoses now subsumed under the rubric of somatoform disorders, with the exception of body dysmorphic disorder which can be placed among the anxiety disorders. Somatic symptoms and syndromes can find room in the third axis of DSM. The advantage of this classification is that it departs from the organic/functional dichotomy of medical disturbances and from the misleading and dangerous assumption that if organic factors cannot be identified, there should be psychiatric reasons which may be able to fully explain the somatic symptomatology. Psychosomatic literature provides an endless series of examples of investigations where psychological factors could only account for part of the unexplained medical disorders [127]. Similarly, the presence of a nonfunctional medical disorder does not exclude, but indeed increases the likelihood of psychological distress and abnormal illness behavior [67].

The diagnostic proposals presented in this chapter will hopefully allow a more specific designation of problems that commonly present to both primary care as well as psychiatric physicians. The current classifications have not advanced our knowledge of such somatic complaints that often have concurrent issues that comprise much of this discussion. In addition, the DCPR will be a unique educational vehicle for all physicians who are woefully ignorant of somatoform disorders, in both classification and management.

Acknowledgements

Supported in part by a grant from the Ministero dell'Università e della Ricerca Scientifica e Tecnologica (MURST, Roma, Italy) to Dr. Fava.

References

1 American Psychiatric Association: Diagnostic and Statistical Manual of Mental disorders, ed 3. Washington, American Psychiatric Association, 1980.
2 Fava GA: The concept of psychosomatic disorder. Psychother Psychosom 1992;58:1–12.
3 Kellner R: Psychosomatic syndromes, somatization and somatoform disorders. Psychother Psychosom 1994;61:4–24.
4 Lipowski ZJ: Somatization. Am J Psychiatry 1987;47:160–167.
5 Mayou R, Kirmayer LJ, Simon G, Kroenke K, Sharpe M: Somatoform disorders: time for a new approach in DSM-V. Am J Psychiatry 2005;162:847–855.
6 Sensky T: Somatization: syndromes or processes? Psychother Psychosom 1994;61:1–3.
7 Wise TN, Birket-Smith TN: The somatoform disorders for DSM-V: the need for changes in process and content. Psychosomatics 2000;43:437–440.
8 Starcevic V: Somatoform disorders and the DSM-V. Psychosomatics 2006;47:277–281.
9 Hiller W, Rief W: Why DSM-III was right to introduce the concept of somatoform disorders. Psychosomatics 2005;46:105–108.
10 Noyes R, Stuart S, Watson DB, Langbehn DR: Distinguishing between hypochondriasis and somatization disorder. Psychother Psychosom 2006;75:270–281.
11 Fava GA, Freyberger HJ, Bech P, Christodoulou G, Sensky T, Theorell T, Wise TN: Diagnostic criteria for use in psychosomatic research. Psychother Psychosom 1995;63;1–8.
12 Pilowsky I: Abnormal Illness Behaviour. Chichester, Wiley, 1997.
13 World Health Organization: The ICD-10 Classification of Mental and Behavioural Disorders. Geneva, World Health Organization, 1992.
14 Beresnevaité M, Taylor GJ, Bagby RM: Assessing alexithymia and type A behavior in coronary heart disease patients: a multimethod approach. Psychother Psychosom 2007;76:186–192.
15 Galeazzi GM, Ferrari S, Mackinnon A, Rigatelli M: Interrater reliability, prevalence and relation to ICD-10 diagnoses of the Diagnostic Criteria for Psychosomatic Research in consultation-liaison psychiatry patients. Psychosomatics 2004;45:386–393.
16 Grandi S, Fabbri S, Tossani E, Mangelli L, Branzi A, Magelli C: Psychological evaluation after cardiac transplantation. Psychother Psychosom 2001;70:176–183.
17 Grassi L, Sabato S, Rossi E, Biancosino B, Marmai L: Use of the Diagnostic Criteria for Psychosomatic Research in oncology. Psychother Psychosom 2005;74:100–107.
18 Mangelli L, Fava GA, Grandi S, Grassi L, Ottolini F, Porcelli P, Rafanelli C, Rigatelli M, Sonino N: Assessing demoralization and depression in the setting of medical disease. J Clin Psychiatry 2005;66:391–394.
19 Mangelli L, Fava GA, Grassi L, Ottolini F, Paolini S, Porcelli P, Rafanelli C, Rigatelli M, Sonino N: Irritable mood in Italian patients with medical disease. J Nerv Ment Dis 2006;194:226–228.
20 Mangelli L, Semprini F, Sirri L, Fava GA, Sonino N: Use of the Diagnostic Criteria for Psychosomatic Research (DCPR) in a community sample. Psychosomatics 2006;47:143–146.
21 Ottolini F, Modena MG, Rigatelli M: Prodromal symptoms in myocardial infarction. Psychother Psychosom 2005;74:323–327.
22 Picardi A, Pasquini P, Abeni D, Fassone G, Mazzotti E, Fava GA: Psychosomatic assessment of skin diseases in clinical practice. Psychother Psychosom 2005;74:315–322.
23 Picardi A, Porcelli P, Pasquini P, Fassone G, Mazzotti E, Lega I, Ramieri L, Sagoni E, Abeni D, Tiago A, Fava GA: Integration of multiple criteria for psychosomatic assessment of dermatological patients. Psychosomatics 2006;47:122–128.

24 Porcelli P, de Carne M, Fava GA: Assessing somatization in functional gastrointestinal disorders Integration of different criteria. Psychother Psychosom 2000;69:198–204.
25 Porcelli P, de Carne M, Todarello O: Prediction of treatment outcome of patients with functional gastrointestinal disorders by the Diagnostic Criteria for Psychosomatic Research. Psychother Psychosom 2004;73:166–173.
26 Rafanelli C, Roncuzzi R, Finos L, Tossani E, Tomba E, Mangelli L, Urbinati S, Pinelli G, Fava GA: Psychosocial assessment in cardiac rehabilitation. Psychother Psychosom 2003;72:343–349.
27 Rafanelli C, Roncuzzi R, Milaneschi Y, Tomba E, Colistro MC, Pancaldi LG, Di Pasquale G: Stressful life events, depression and demoralization as risk factors for acute coronary heart disease. Psychother Psychosom 2005;74:179–184.
28 Rafanelli C, Roncuzzi R, Milaneschi Y: Minor depression as a cardiac risk factor after coronary artery bypass surgery. Psychosomatics 2006;47:289–295.
29 Sonino N, Navarrini C, Ruini C, Ottolini F, Paoletta A, Fallo F, Boscaro M, Fava GA: Persistent psychological distress in patients treated for endocrine disease. Psychother Psychosom 2004;73:78–83.
30 Sonino N, Fallo F, Fava GA: Psychological aspects of primary aldosteronism. Psychother Psychosom 2006;75:327–330.
31 Fukunishi I, Hosaka T, Aoki T, Azekawa T, Ota A, Miyaoka H: Criterion-related validity of diagnostic criteria for alexithymia in a general hospital psychiatric setting. Psychother Psychosom 1996;65:82–85.
32 Littman AB: Review of psychosomatic aspects of cardiovascular disease. Psychother Psychosom 1993;60:148–167.
33 Kellner R: Somatization and Hypochondriasis. New York, Praeger, 1986.
34 Kellner R: Abridged Manual of the Illness Attitude Scale. Albuquerque, Universtity of New Mexico, 1987.
35 Kellner R, Abbott P, Winslow WW, Pathak D: Fears, beliefs, and attitudes in DSM-III hypochondriasis. J Nerv Ment Dis 1987;175:20–25.
36 Fava GA, Grandi S: Differential diagnosis of hypochondriacal fears and beliefs. Psychother Psychosom 1991;55:114–119.
37 Bartolucci G, Savron G, Fava GA, Grandi S, Trombini G, Orlandi C: Psychological reactions in thermography and mammography. Stress Med 1989;5:195–199.
38 Ryle JA: Angor animi, or the sense of dying. Guys Hosp Rep 1928;78:230–235.
39 Fava GA, Kellner R, Zielenzy M, Grandi S: Hypochondriacal fears and beliefs in agoraphobia. J Affect Disord 1988;14:239–244.
40 Fava GA, Grandi S, Saviotti FM, Conti S: Hypochondriasis with panic attacks. Psychosomatics 1990;31:351–353.
41 Morselli E: Sulla dismorfofobia e sulla tafefobia. Boll Reale Accad Med Genova 1891;6:5–14.
42 Mayer-Gross W, Slater E, Roth M: Clinical Psychiatry. London, Doilliere Tindall, 1969.
43 Bianchi GN: Origins of disease phobia. Aust N Z J Psychiatry 1971;5:241–257.
44 Ryle JA: Nosophobia. Br J Psychiatry 1948;94:1–17.
45 Conti S, Savron G, Bartolucci G, Grandi S, Magelli C, Semprini F, Saviotti FM, Trombini G, Fava GA, Magnani B: Cardiac neurosis and psychopathology. Psychother Psychosom 1989;52: 88–91.
46 Noyes R, Carney CP, Langbehn DR: Specific phobia of illness: search for a new subtype. J Anxiety Disord 2004;18:531–545.
47 Pilowsky I: Dimensions of hypochondriasis. Br J Psychiatry 1967;113:89–93.
48 Warwick HMC, Marks IM: Behavioural treatment of illness phobia and hypochondriasis. Br J Psychiatry 1998;152:239–241.
49 Wesner RB, Noyes R: Imipramine an effective treatment for illness phobia. J Affect Disord 1991;22:43–48.
50 Freud A: The Ego and the Mechanisms of Defense. London, Hogarth, 1961.
51 Lazarus RS: The costs and benefits of denial; in Breznitz S (ed): The Denial of Stress. New York, International Universities Press, 1983.
52 Goldbeck R: Denial in physical illness. J Psychosom Res 1997;43:575–593.
53 Breznitz S: The seven kinds of denial; in Breznitz S (ed): The Denial of Stress. New York, International Universities Press, 1983.

54 Garay-Sevilla ME, Malacara JM, Gutiérrez-Roa A, Gonzalez E: Denial of disease in Type 2 diabetes mellitus: its influence on metabolic control and associated factors. Diabetic Med 1999;16: 238–244.
55 Kreitler S: Denial in cancer patients. Cancer Invest 1999;17:514–534.
56 Young LD, Schweiger J, Beitzinger J, McManus R, Bloedel C, Koob J: Denial in heart transplant candidates. Psychother Psychosom 1991;55:141–144.
57 Ben-Zur H, Breznitz S, Wardi N, Berzon Y: Denial of HIV/AIDS and preventive behaviour among Israeli adolescents. J Adolesc 2000;23:157–174.
58 American Psychiatric Association: Diagnostic and Statistical Manual of Mental Disorders, ed 4. Washington, American Psychiatric Association, 1994.
59 Appelbaum PS: Why denial of physical illness is not a 'diagnosis'. Int J Psychiatry Med 1998;28: 479–482.
60 Muskin PR, Feldhammer T, Gelfand JL, Strauss DH: Maladaptive denial of physical illness: a useful new 'diagnosis'. Int J Psychiatry Med 1998;28:463–477.
61 Strauss DH, Spitzer RL, Muskin PR: Maladaptive denial of physical illness: a proposal for DSM-IV. Am J Psychiatry 1990;147:1168–1172.
62 Creed F, Barsky AA: Systematic review of the epidemiology of somatization disorder and hypochondriasis. J Psychosom Res 2004;56:391–408.
63 Kroenke K, Swindle R: Cognitive-behavioral therapy for somatization and symptom syndromes: a critical review of controlled clinical trials. Psychother Psychosom 2000;69:205–215.
64 Stone J, Smyth R, Carson A, Lewis S, Prescott R, Warlow C, Sharpe M: Systematic review of misdiagnosis of conversion symptoms and 'hysteria'. BMJ 2005;331:989.
65 Engel GL: Conversion symptoms; in MacBryde CM, Blacklow RS (eds): Signs and Symptoms. Philadelphia, Lippincott, 1970, pp 650–669.
66 Stone J, Smyth R, Carson A, Warlow C, Sharpe M: La belle indifférence in conversion symptoms and hysteria. Br J Psychiatry 2006;188:204–209.
67 Lipowski ZJ: Physical illness and psychopathology. Int J Psychiatry Med 1974;5:483–497.
68 Daie N, Witztum E: Short-term strategic treatment in traumatic conversion reaction. Am J Psychother 1991;45:335–347.
69 Diseth TH, Christie HJ: Trauma-related dissociative (conversion) disorders in children and adolescents – an overview of assessment tools and treatment principles. Nord J Psychiatr 2005;59: 278–292.
70 Krull F, Schifferdeker M: Inpatient treatment of conversion disorder: a clinical investigation of outcome. Psychother Psychosom 1990;53:161–165.
71 Wald J, Taylor S, Scamvougeras A: Cognitive behavioural and neuropsychiatric treatment of post-traumatic conversion disorder: a case study. Cogn Behav Ther 2004;33:12–20.
72 Fava GA, Magelli C, Savron G, Conti S, Bartolucci G, Grandi S, Semptini F, Saviotti FM, Belluardo P, Magnani B: Neurocirculatory asthenia. Acta Psychiatr Scand 1994;89:314–319.
73 Kellner R: Psychosomatic Syndromes and Somatic Symptoms. Washington, American Psychiatric Press, 1991.
74 Engel GL: The death of a twin. Int J Psychoanal 1975;56:23–40.
75 Hilgard JR: Anniversary reactions in parents precipitated by children. Psychiatry 1953;16:73–80.
76 Hilgard JR, Newman MF: Anniversaries in mental illness. Psychiatry 1959;22:113–121.
77 Chapman AH: The concept of nemesis in psychoneurosis. J Nerv Ment Dis 1959;129:29–34.
78 Frank JD: Psychotherapy: the restoration of morale. Am J Psychiatry 1974;131:271–274.
79 Frank JD, Frank JB: Persuasion and Healing: a Comparative Study of Psychotherapy. Baltimore, Johns Hopkins University Press, 1993.
80 Slavney PR: Diagnosing demoralization in consultation psychiatry. Psychosomatics 1999;40: 325–329.
81 Dohrenwend BP, Shrout PE, Egri G, Mendelsohn FS: Nonspecific psychological distress and other dimensions of psychopathology. Arch Gen Psychiatry 1980;37:1229–1236.
82 de Figueiredo JM: Depression and demoralization: phenomenologic differences and research perspectives. Compr Psychiatry 1993;34:308–311.
83 Schmale AH, Engel GL: The giving up-given up complex illustrated on film. Arch Gen Psychiatry 1967;17:133–145.

84 Clarke DM, Kissane DW: Demoralization: its phenomenology and importance. Aust N Z J Psychiatry 2002;36:733–742.
85 Grossarth-Maticek R, Bastiaans J, Kanazir DT: Psychosocial factors as strong predictors of mortality from cancer, ischaemic heart disease and stroke: the Yugoslav prospective study. J Psychosom Res 1985;29:167–176.
86 Schuitemaker GE, Dinant GJ, van der Pol GA, Appels A: Assessment of vital exhaustion and identification of subjects at increased risk of myocardial infarction in general practice. Psychosomatics 2004;45:414–418.
87 Beck AT, Weissman A, Lester D, Trexler L: The measurement of pessimism: the hopelessness scale. J Consult Clin Psychol 1974;42:861–865.
88 Clarke DM, Smith GC, Dowe DL, McKenzie DP: An empirically derived taxonomy of common distress syndromes in the medically ill. J Psychosom Res 2003;54:323–330.
89 Feldman D, Rabinowitz J, Yehuda YB: Detecting psychological distress among patients attending secondary health care clinics. Gen Hosp Psychiatry 1995;17:425–432.
90 Snaith RP, Taylor CM: Irritability. Br J Psychiatry 1985;147:127–136.
91 Fava GA: Irritable mood and physical illness. Stress Med 1987;3:293–299.
92 Fava M: Depression with anger attacks. J Clin Psychiatry 1998;59:18–22.
93 Fava GA, Grandi S, Rafanelli C, Saviotti FM, Ballin M, Pesarin F: Hostility and irritable mood in panic disorder with agoraphobia. J Affect Disord 1993;29:213–217.
94 Winkler D, Pjrek E, Kasper S: Anger attacks in depression – evidence for a male depressive syndrome. Psychother Psychosom 2005;74:303–307.
95 Fava GA: Affective disorders and endocrine disease. New insights from psychosomatic studies. Psychosomatics 1994;35:341–353.
96 Miller TQ, Smith TW, Turner CW, Guijarro ML, Hallet AJ: A meta-analytic review of research on hostility and physical health. Psychol Bull 1996;119:322–348.
97 Eaker ED, Sullivan LM, Kelly-Hayes M, D'Agostino RB, Benjamin EJ: Anger and hostility predict the development of atrial fibrillation in men in the Framingham Offspring Study. Circulation 2004;109:1267–1271.
98 Ketterer MW, Mahr G, Goldberg AD: Psychological factors affecting a medical condition: ischemic coronary heart disease. J Psychosom Res 2000;48:357–367.
99 Bennett EJ, Piesse C, Palmer K, Badcock CA, Tennant CC, Kellow JE: Functional gastrointestinal disorders: psychological, social, and somatic features. Gut 1998;42:414–420.
100 Fukunishi I, Hosaka T, Rahe RH: Are abnormal gastrofiberscopic findings related to hostility with poor social support or to negative responses to stress? J Psychosom Res 1996;41:337–342.
101 Welgan P, Meshkinpour H, Ma L: Role of anger in antral motor activity in irritable bowel syndrome. Dig Dis Sci 2000;45:248–251.
102 Miller TQ, Markides KS, Chiriboga DA, Ray LA: A test of the psychosocial vulnerability and health behavior models of hostility: results from an 11-year follow-up study of Mexican Americans. Psychosom Med 1995;57:572–581.
103 Friedman M, Rosenman RH: Association of specific overt behavior pattern with blood and cardiovascular findings. JAMA 1959;169:1286–1295.
104 Friedman M, Rosenman RH: Type A Behavior and Your Heart. New York, Knopf, 1974.
105 Fava M, Littman A, Halperin P: Neuroendocrine correlates of the type A behavior pattern: a review and new hypotheses. Int J Psychiatry Med 1987;17:289–307.
106 Rosenman RH, Brand RJ, Jenkins CD, Friedman M, Straus R, Wurm M: Coronary heart disease in the Western Collaborative Group Study: final follow-up experience of 85 years. JAMA 1975;233:872–877.
107 Haynes S, Feinleib M, Levine S, Scotch N, Kannel W: The relationship of psychosocial factors to coronary heart disease in the Framingham Study: prevalence of coronary heart disease. Am J Epidemiol 1978;107:384–389.
108 Cole SR, Kawachi I, Liu S, Gaziano JM, Manson JE, Buring JE, Hennekens CH: Time urgency and risk of non-fatal myocardial infarction. Int J Epidemiol 2001;30:363–369.
109 Friedman M: Type A Behavior: Its Diagnosis and Treatment. New York, Plenum Press, 1996.
110 Sparagon B, Friedman M, Breall WS, Goodwin ML, Fleischmann N, Ghandour G: Type A behavior and coronary atherosclerosis. Atherosclerosis 2001;156:145–149.

111 Jenkins CD, Rosenman RH: Development of an objective test for the determination of the coronary-prone behavior pattern in employed men. J Chronic Dis 1967;20:371–379.
112 Ornish D, Brown SE, Scherwitz LW, Billings JH, Armstrong WT, Ports TA, McLanahan SM, Kirkeeide RL, Brand RJ, Gould KL: Can lifestyle changes reverse coronary heart disease? Lancet 1990;336:129–133.
113 Ornish D, Scherwitz LW, Billings JH, Gould KL, Merritt TA, Sparler S, Armstrong WT, Ports TA, Kirkeeide RL, Hogeboom C, Brand RJ: Intensive lifestyle changes for reversal of coronary heart disease. JAMA 1998;280:2001–2007.
114 Sebregts EH, Falger PR, Bar FW: Risk factor modification through nonpharmacological interventions in patients with coronary heart disease. J Psychosom Res 2000;48:425–441.
115 Michaelsen A, Grossman P, Lehmann N, Knoblauch NTM, Paul A, Moebius S, Buddle T, Dobos GJ: Psychological and quality-of-life outcomes from a comprehensive stress reduction and lifestyle program in patients with coronary artery disease. Psychother Psychosom 2005;74:344–352.
116 Sifneos PE: The prevalence of alexithymic characteristics in psychosomatic patients. Psychother Psychosom 1973;22:255–262.
117 Sifneos PE: Affect, emotional conflict, and deficit: an overview. Psychother Psychosom 1991;56: 116–122.
118 Porcelli P, Taylor GJ, Bagby RM, De Carne M: Alexithymia and functional gastrointestinal disorder. Psychother Psychosom 1999;68:263–269.
119 Bach M, Bach D: Alexithymia in somatoform disorders and somatic diseases. Psychother Psychosom 1996;65:150–152.
120 Honkalampi K, Saarinen P, Hintikka J, Virtanen V, Viinamaki H: Factors associated with alexithymia in patients suffering from depression. Psychother Psychosom 1999;68:270–275.
121 Iancu I, Horesh N, Offer D, Dannon PN, Lepkifker E, Kotler M: Alexithymia, affect intensity and emotional range in suicidal patients. Psychother Psychosom 1999;68:276–280.
122 Berenbaum H, Davis R, McGrew J: Alexithymia and the interpretation of hostile-provoking situations. Psychother Psychosom 1998;67:254–258.
123 Kooiman CG, Spinhoven P, Truiisburg RW, Roojmans HGM: Perceived parental attitude, alexithymia and defense style in psychiatric outpatients. Psychother Psychosom 1998;67:81–87.
124 Taylor GJ: Recent developments in alexithymia theory and research. Can J Psychiatry 2000;45: 134–142.
125 Lumley MA, Stettner L, Wehmer F: How are alexithymia and physical illness linked? A review and critique of pathways. J Psychosom Res 1996;41:505–518.
126 Kissen DM: The significance of syndrome shift and late syndrome association in psychosomatic medicine. J Nerv Ment Dis 1963;136:34–42.
127 Fava GA, Sonino N: The clinical domains of psychosomatic medicine. J Clin Psychiatry 2005;66:849–858.
128 Halliday JL: The significance of the concept of a psychosomatic affection. Psychosom Med 1945;7:240–245.
129 Fava GA: A different medicine is possible. Psychother Psychosom 2006;75:1–3.
130 Fava GA, Fabbri S, Sirri L, Wise TN: Psychological factors affecting medical condition: a new proposal for DSM-V. Psychosomatics 2007;48:103–111.

Giovanni A. Fava, MD
Department of Psychology, University of Bologna
Viale Berti Pichat 5
IT–40127 Bologna (Italy)
Tel. +39 051 209 1339, Fax +39 051 243 086, E-Mail giovanniandrea.fava@unibo.it

Porcelli P, Sonino N (eds): Psychological Factors Affecting Medical Conditions. A New Classification for DSM-V. Adv Psychosom Med. Basel, Karger, 2007, vol 28, pp 21–33

Psychosocial Approach to Endocrine Disease

Nicoletta Sonino[a,c], *Elena Tomba*[b], *Giovanni A. Fava*[b,c]

[a]Departments of Statistical Sciences and Mental Health, University of Padova, Padova, and [b]Department of Psychology, University of Bologna, Bologna, Italy; [c]Department of Psychiatry, State University of New York at Buffalo, Buffalo, N.Y., USA

Abstract

In recent years, there has been growing interest in the psychosocial aspects of endocrine disease, such as the role of life stress in the pathogenesis of some conditions, their association with affective disorders, and the presence of residual symptoms after adequate treatment. In clinical endocrinology, exploration of psychosocial antecedents may elucidate the temporal relationships between life events and symptom onset, as it has been shown to be relevant for pituitary (Cushing's disease, hyperprolactinemia) or thyroid (Graves' disease) conditions, as well as the role of allostatic load, linked to chronic stress, in uncovering a person's vulnerability. After endocrine abnormalities are established, they are frequently associated with a wide range of psychological symptoms: at times, such symptoms reach the level of psychiatric illness (mainly mood and anxiety disorders); at other times, however, they can only be identified by the subclinical forms of assessment provided by the Diagnostic Criteria for Psychosomatic Research (DCPR). Indeed, in a population study, the majority of patients suffered from at least one of the three DCPR syndromes considered: irritable mood, demoralization, persistent somatization. In particular, irritable mood was found to occur in 46% of 146 patients successfully treated for endocrine conditions, a rate similar to that found in cardiology and higher than in oncology and gastroenterology. Long-standing endocrine disorders may imply a degree of irreversibility of the pathological process and induce highly individualized affective responses. In patients who showed persistence or even worsening of psychological distress upon proper endocrine treatment, the value of appropriate psychiatric interventions was underscored. As it happened in other fields of clinical medicine, a conceptual shift from a merely biomedical care to a psychosomatic consideration of the person and his/her quality of life appears to be necessary for improving effectiveness in endocrinology. The DCPR have been demonstrated to be a valuable tool for psychological assessment in the various phases of endocrine disease from diagnostic to follow-up periods.

In recent years, there has been growing interest in the psychosocial aspects of endocrine disease. A number of studies have documented important morbidity and impaired quality of life in patients with various forms of endocrine disease [1–3]. Moreover, psychological distress was found to persist even with cured, or acceptably compensated, endocrine disorders of different kinds [4]. Patients have become more aware of these issues. Their difficulties in coping with endocrine illness and its often severe psychiatric consequences have indeed led to the development of several patients' associations in recent years. As the issues of psychological well-being, functional capacity, and social and interpersonal components of medical illness are further developing [5], the domain of quality of life may provide new insights also into clinical endocrinology. Research evidence for an updated psychosocial comprehension of endocrine disease is available. We will try to highlight some of the areas in endocrinology where the psychosocial aspects of illness may have important clinical and research implications.

Psychosocial Antecedents

Short-term acute, experimental stress has become the focus of a large volume of endocrine research, but the validity of laboratory stressors as models for those of real life has been questioned, and the extension and applicability of laboratory results to long-term situations is purely inferential [6, 7]. Nonetheless, many kinds of psychological stress, both acute and chronic, in experimental or real-life situations, have been shown to involve the hypothalamic-pituitary-adrenal axis. Psychological factors may either raise or lower the level of pituitary-adrenal activity. The outcome is the result of important variables including the quality of emotional reaction, the style and effectiveness of psychological defenses, and whether the threat is of an acute or chronic nature [6, 7]. Chronic stress incorporates several elements, including life events. By 'life events' are meant discrete changes in the subject's social or personal environment, that should be external and verifiable rather than internal or psychological. They may play a substantial role in uncovering a person's vulnerability to a particular physical or psychiatric disorder [8]. By structured methods of data collection and control groups, this has been demonstrated for some endocrine conditions, confirming clinical observations scattered throughout the literature.

Several intriguing issues have emerged in studying Cushing's syndrome. Stressful life events in the year before the first signs of disease onset were investigated by Paykel's Interview for Recent Life Events [8] in 66 consecutive patients with Cushing's syndrome of various etiologies and in 66 healthy subjects matched for sociodemographic variables [9]. The patients with Cushing's syndrome reported significantly more losses, undesirable events and uncontrolled events than controls. The results did not depend on the well-known relationship between life events and depression, since there were no differences between patients with and without major depression. When patients with pituitary-dependent Cushing's disease and patients with pituitary-independent Cushing's syndrome (primary adrenal hyperfunction and ectopic ACTH production) were evaluated separately and compared with their matched controls, a causal role for stressful life events was found exclusively in Cushing's disease [9], supporting the hypothesis of a limbic-hypothalamic involvement in the pathogenesis of this condition [10].

By the same rigorous method employed for Cushing's syndrome, life events have been investigated in 70 consecutive patients with Graves' disease and found to be significantly more frequent than in controls [11]. The same conclusions were drawn by different studies: by mailing a questionnaire about life changes to 219 patients with Graves' disease and 372 control subjects [12]; by a self-reporting questionnaire recalling life events, daily stress and coping in 95 patients compared to their matched controls [13], and by using Paykel's Interview for Recent Life Events in 100 newly diagnosed patients with Graves' disease and 100 controls [14]. Stressful life events may affect the regulatory mechanism of immune function in a number of ways [5, 7, 15]. Within the complex pathogenesis of autoimmune thyroid hyperfunction, these studies, as well as several clinical uncontrolled observations, emphasize the role of emotional stress.

Life events, using Paykel's scale [8], have also been investigated in 52 consecutive patients with hyperprolactinemia and found to be significantly more frequent than in controls [16]. There were no significant differences between patients with prolactinoma and those with idiopathic hyperprolactinemia. The findings lend support to previous investigations suggesting that early adverse experiences may influence hormone patterns in later life. Indeed, exposure during childhood to an environment characterized by an absent or alcoholic, violent father may condition some women to develop hyperprolactinemia and/or galactorrhea later in life as a response to specific environmental changes, such as marriage or actual or threatened loss of an important person [17]. Accordingly, both entrances and exits from the social field were reported significantly more frequently by hyperprolactinemic patients compared to controls [16].

Life changes are not the only source of psychological stress. Subtle and longstanding life situations should not too readily be dismissed as minor and negligible, since chronic, daily life stresses may be appraised by the individual as taxing or exceeding his or her coping skills. McEwen and Stellar [18, 19] suggested a formulation of the relationship between stress and the processes leading to disease, based on the concept of allostasis, the ability of the organism to achieve stability through change. They propose that 'through allostasis, the autonomic nervous system, the hypothalamic-pituitary-adrenal axis, and the cardiovascular, metabolic and immune systems protect the body by responding to internal and external stress' [19]. The allostatic load is the cost of chronic exposure to fluctuating or heightened neural or neuroendocrine response resulting from repeated or chronic environmental challenge that an individual reacts to as being particularly stressful. It emphasizes the hidden burden of chronic stress on the body over long periods of time [18, 19].

The psychoneuroendocrine balance between health and disease may be affected by allostatic load exceeding personal resources [20, 21]. Patients with endocrine disorders displayed significantly higher levels of allostatic load, as measured by the Psychosocial Index [22], compared to controls [23]. The allostatic load was significantly more pronounced in endocrine patients who also suffered from psychiatric illness or psychological clusters identified by the Diagnostic Criteria for Psychosomatic Research (DCPR) [4].

In clinical endocrinology, exploration of psychosocial antecedents may thus elucidate the following. (a) Temporal relationships between life events and symptom onset or relapse. (b) Presence of grief reactions, including the loss of a body part or bodily function. Gradual changes which occur with chronic progressive disease may give the individual time to perceive and tolerate the changes, whereas sudden modifications are potentially more disruptive and grief inducing [5]. (c) Perception of an environment by the person as exceeding his/her resources (allostatic load). Often patients deny a relationship between their allostatic load and symptomatology, since they are unaware of the latency between stress accumulation and symptom onset. Symptomatic worsening during week-ends and vacation time is a common manifestation of this latency. This information may be crucial in assessing patients with borderline laboratory findings (e.g. slightly elevated prolactin levels).

In our clinical experience, the suggestion of lifestyle modifications may considerably improve mild hormonal alterations linked to allostatic load. Further, appraisal of life stress may have important implications for clinical decisions, such as termination of the long-term pharmacological treatment in hyperprolactinemia [16], and in the presence of unexplained somatic symptoms or delayed recovery [2].

Psychological Aspects

Endocrine disorders may be associated with a wide range of psychological symptoms. At times, such symptoms reach the level of psychiatric illness, mainly mood and anxiety disorders [2], as listed in table 1. At other times, however, psychiatric nosography fails to capture psychological distress and this can

Table 1. Endocrine disorders associated with high psychiatric morbidity

Endocrine disorder	Psychiatric characteristics
Cushing's syndrome	Major depression is a life-threatening complication which may affect 50–60% of patients. It occurs in both pituitary dependent and -independent forms Antidepressants are often ineffective, while inhibitors of steroid production are generally effective. Anxiety is frequently present. At times, mania may alternate with depression [27]
Addison's disease	Depression (characterized by apathy, negativism, social withdrawal and irritability) is often present and generally responsive to steroid replacement [54, 55]
Primary aldosteronism	It is particularly associated with anxiety disorders [32]
Hyperthyroidism	Major depression (often associated with anxiety and irritability) is the most common complication. It is generally responsive to adequate endocrine treatment. Sometimes, antidepressant drugs are required [54, 55]
Hypothyroidism	Depression, paranoid disorder, and severe cognitive disturbances may occur. At times they may persist even after appropriate treatment [54, 55]
Hyperprolactinemia	Depression, hostility and anxiety are common. Bromocriptine was found to be superior to placebo, while antidepressant drugs were ineffective [37, 38, 54]
Hyperparathyroidism	It may be associated with a variety of psychiatric alterations, particularly in women [55]

only be identified by the use of forms of assessment for subclinical symptoms, such as the DCPR [24]. Indeed, in an investigation on 146 patients treated for endocrine disease, 62% presented at least one psychiatric diagnosis, whereas 66% suffered from at least one of the three DCPR syndromes considered (demoralization, irritable mood, persistent somatization). Eighty-one percent of the patients presented with either a psychiatric or psychological (DCPR) diagnosis. About one fifth of the patients had a DCPR cluster only. We will briefly describe the main psychological correlates of endocrine disease, including both DSM-IV (table 1) and DCPR (table 2) syndromes. At times, psychological symptoms may precede other manifestations of an endocrine disorder and/or be early indicators of its relapse [25].

Depression

Depressive symptoms are frequently encountered in the medically ill [26]. However, only a limited number of patients suffer from a major depressive

Table 2. Endocrine disorders associated with DCPR psychological clusters

Endocrine disorder	Psychological characteristics
Cushing's syndrome	Demoralization and irritable mood are common both in the acute phase of illness and in the phase of recovery, particularly when the latter is delayed [4, 27]
Primary aldosteronism	Demoralization is frequently reported in conjunction with anxiety [32]
Hyperthyroidism	Irritability is very common [33] and is often associated with anxiety and depression. It may persist after normalization of thyroid hormone levels [4]
Hyperprolactinemia	Hostility and irritable mood are frequently present and may persist in some cases with normalization of prolactin levels, together with persistent somatization and demoralization [4, 34–38]

disorder, that is depressed mood associated with loss of interest or pleasure, appetite changes, sleep disturbances, psychomotor retardation or agitation, fatigue, feelings of worthlessness and guilt, suicidal thoughts. When depression is associated with a physical disorder, the potential relationships in the development of the mood disturbance range from a purely coincidental occurrence to a direct causal role of organic factors. The latter is subsumed under the rubric of symptomatic depression or organic mood disorder, whose key feature is the resolution of psychiatric disturbances upon specific treatment of the organic disease [26]. Symptomatic depressions are commonly associated with endocrine disorders (table 1), and among them mainly with Cushing's syndrome [27]. In many physical diseases (e.g. myocardial infarction), the presence of depression was found to connote an unfavorable prognosis [5]. Similarly, in pituitary-dependent Cushing's disease, the presence of depression was found to be associated with severity of clinical presentation as well as to entail prognostic value. Indeed, patients were more likely to relapse after successful pituitary microadenomectomy if they presented with depression [28].

Mania

The occurrence of mania, a distinct period of abnormally and persistently elevated and expansive mood (with symptoms such as grandiosity, decreased need to sleep, distractibility, increase in goal-directed activity, excessive involvement in pleasurable activities, pressure to keep talking and flight of ideas), is much less frequent than that of depression in the medically ill [25, 27]. In Cushing's syndrome, manic or hypomanic symptoms may however take place and be among the early manifestations of illness [25, 27]. They are rare in other endocrine disorders, and may occur as a complication of drug therapy, such as during treatment of hypothyroidism with high-dose thyroid replacement [29].

Anxiety

Anxiety, a fearful anticipation of an imminent but intangible danger, may be related to endocrine illness in a number of ways. It may occur as recurrent, prominent attacks or as generalized anxiety. One should exclude the presence of a major depressive disorder, in which case anxiety symptoms may be part of the symptomatology (as frequently appears to be the case in Cushing's syndrome). As with depression, when anxiety disorders are associated with a medical illness, the potential relationship ranges from a coincidental occurrence to a direct causal role of hormone imbalances. The relationship of anxiety to hyperthyroidism exemplifies this controversial aspect. Anxiety disorders may be precipitated by hyperthyroidism and may abate with its treatment, but may also antedate its clinical manifestations or predispose to its onset [30]. Pheochromocytoma is associated with anxiety symptoms, which however do not satisfy the criteria for a psychiatric anxiety disorder, such as panic disorder or generalized anxiety [31]. An association between anxiety disorders (mainly generalized anxiety disorder) and primary aldosteronism has been recently reported [32].

Irritability

Irritability has been associated with several endocrine disorders. A survey of neuropsychiatric complaints of 137 patients with Graves' disease [33] found that it was the most frequent symptom, occurring in nearly 80% of patients. In hyperprolactinemia, in a number of independent studies using different methods of assessment [34–37], hostility and irritable mood were consistently reported in women (independently of depression) and were responsive to lowering of plasma prolactin levels by bromocriptine but not to placebo [38]. In the medical setting, irritability is often dismissed as an understandable reaction to hospitalization, pain and diagnostic procedures. However, it becomes a condition worthy of clinical attention when it is characterized by a prolonged and generalized state, with difficult control over temper, or by angry-explosive attacks that are egodystonic to the patient, as described in the DCPR [24]. Irritable mood was found to occur in 46% of 146 patients who had been successfully treated for endocrine disease [4]. This indicates that it may persist after normalization of endocrine parameters and lead to considerable strain on the patients' interactions with others. In a study comparing irritable mood in a variety of medical conditions [39], it was significantly more prevalent in cardiology and endocrinology, compared to oncology and gastroenterology.

Demoralization

The DCPR identify a syndrome characterized by the patient's consciousness of having failed to meet his or her own expectations or those of others or being unable to cope with some pressing problems. Schmale and Engel [40] have provided a detailed account of demoralization, which they defined as the 'giving up-given up complex'. It involves distressing feelings ascribed by the patient at times more to failures and deficiencies in his/her environment (helplessness) and at times more to his/her own personal failures and inadequacies for which he/she feels nothing can be done (hopelessness). The patient perceives himself/herself as less competent and less in control [40]. In the various phases of endocrine diseases (the frequent long interval from the appearance of the first symptoms to a proper diagnosis, the period for endocrine work-up which may be lengthy and fatiguing, the long time required to recover after surgery or radiotherapy), there are important sources of demoralization. Demoralization according to the DCPR [24] was found to occur in about one third of remitted endocrine patients, with rates similar to those which were found after myocardial infarction or heart transplantation and in oncology [41]. Sometimes demoralization may occur in conjunction with major depression, but in most of the cases it is independent [41].

Persistent Somatization

Somatization is defined by Lipowski [42] as the tendency to experience and communicate psychological distress in the form of physical symptoms and to seek medical help for them.

The DCPR criteria for persistent somatization identify patients in whom psychophysiological symptoms have clustered [24]. These functional symptoms may occur in conjunction with endocrine disturbances and may aggravate the clinical picture. In a sample of 146 patients with remitted endocrine disorders, persistent somatization was found to occur in about one patient out of 5 [4].

Impaired Quality of Life

Psychiatric and psychological variables may have profound effect on the quality of life of patients with endocrine disease.

The concept of quality of life subscribes to the psychosomatic postulate that mind and body are two inseparably linked aspects of man. As Lipowski [43] remarked, 'how a person experiences the pathological process, what it means to him, and how this meaning influences his behavior and interaction with others are all integral components of disease viewed as a total human response'. Functional capacity (the abilities to perform activities of daily life, social interactions, intellectual and cognitive function, and economic status), perceptions (levels of well-being and illness attitudes) and effects of symptoms of disease (with resulting impairment) are thus the main areas of investigation in quality of life research [5]. Psychiatric symptoms, particularly depression, may have a profound influence on quality of life and on how the endocrine disease process is experienced. However, psychological well-being is not simply lack of psychiatric distress (even though it may be influenced by it) and was found to correlate poorly with objective severity of disease [44]. Further, lack of significant psychopathology according to DSM or of specific psychological clusters (DCPR) cannot be equated to an absence of compromised quality of life. For instance, significant psychiatric or psychological disorders were not found in acromegaly, and yet these patients display considerable impairment in self-esteem, body image distortion, disruption in interpersonal relationships, and social withdrawal [45]. Quality of life research in endocrinology has particularly focused on conditions of growth hormone deficiency, and the profound psychological implications of growth hormone deficiency in childhood (disturbances in identity formation, social withdrawal, impaired self-esteem, distorted body image) have long been emphasized [46]. A state of functional growth hormone deficiency in childhood may occur as a result of disruption of social relationships in the neonatal environment. The syndrome, known as psychosocial dwarfism or abuse dwarfism, is characterized by delayed physical, intellectual and emotional growth, and normalizes rapidly with improvement of psychosocial environment [47]. Further, Uhde [47] has postulated a link between growth hormone and anxiety disorders, and particularly social phobia, during development. He raised the possibility that the presence of anxiety disorders in some children, independent of physical or emotional abuse, might produce a growth hormone deficiency that results in clinically meaningful impairment in stature or growth acceleration. Conversely, growth hormone deficiency may be associated with an increased risk of developing an anxiety disorder.

The attention to the compromised quality of life of adults with growth hormone deficiency has been more recent. These patients were found to have difficulties leading a normal professional and private life. They reported social isolation, low interest in pleasurable activities, sexual and cognitive dysfunctions, fatigue and irritability [46]. Such deficiencies have led to the development of a specific quality of life model for adults with growth hormone deficiency [48]. Significant psychological improvement upon recombinant growth hormone was reported in double-blind, placebo-controlled studies [46] and led to the hypothesis of a central growth hormone effect [49].

Psychological Aspects of Management

A treatment primarily directed to the physical condition may be more effective than psychotropic drugs in organic affective syndromes associated with endocrine disease. Examples are provided by the favorable effects of steroid synthesis inhibitors (i.e. metyrapone and ketoconazole) upon depression in Cushing's syndrome and of antithyroid agents on anxiety in hyperthyroidism. Clinical endocrinologists may, thus, tend to underestimate psychiatric symptoms as readily suppressible by adequate medical or surgical treatment. However, disappearance of psychiatric symptoms upon proper endocrine treatment is not always the case. In our experience and in other investigations using definite diagnostic criteria for depression, about 70% of patients fully recovered from their depression after successful treatment of Cushing's syndrome, whereas there were no substantial changes in the others or even worsening in some [50]. In those who actually deteriorated, the value of appropriate psychiatric intervention was underscored. Of interest is the case of a patient in remission from Cushing's syndrome, who responded to an antidepressant drug she had been exposed to unsuccessfully while being hypercortisolemic. Similarly, while phobias and hyperthyroidism frequently coexist, and detection and treatment of hyperthyroidism may also solve patients' long-standing agoraphobia [51], successful management of thyroid hyperfunction is not always sufficient to overcome an anxiety disorder. Since anxiety itself may increase a person's vulnerability to hyperthyroidism, it is important to assess the coexistence of phobias and hyperthyroidism on an individual basis.

Establishing etiological priorities in affective disorders associated with endocrine disease is a complex task that requires considerable clinical skills, and becomes necessary when the patient responds only partially to ongoing appropriate treatment. On the other hand, long-standing endocrine disorders may imply a degree of irreversibility of the pathological process and induce highly individualized affective responses based on each patient's psychological assets and liabilities. Unrealistic hopes of 'cure' may foster demoralization and apathy. For example, when surgery is performed in Cushing's disease (usually pituitary microadenomectomy), the patient is likely to have expectations of a quick recovery to his/her former normal condition. This is seldom the case and patients should be advised that recovery is a lengthy process, even when all different problems are properly addressed [27]. Quality of life may often be seriously compromised also when the patient is apparently doing fine (by a hormonal viewpoint). Research on quality of life has frequently emphasized the discrepancies in health perceptions between patients, their companions and their treating physicians [5]. In clinical endocrinology, there is often the tendency to rely exclusively on 'hard data', preferably expressed in the dimensional numbers of laboratory measurements, excluding 'soft information', such as disability and well-being. This soft information can now, however, be reliably assessed [5, 48]. The evidence that has accumulated on treatment of growth hormone deficiency should lead endocrinologists to a multidimensional assessment of treatment effects, encompassing also psychosocial parameters. For instance, the differential effects on quality of life that are entailed by different doses and/or schedules of replacement therapy are frequently acknowledged in the newsletters of patients' associations, but have received only scanty research attention [2, 52].

Conclusions

As outlined with a few examples, the interrelationship between hormone abnormalities and psychological factors is complex and should be viewed in a multifactorial frame of reference. A first simple implication would be for the clinician to be reminded of 'the necessity for the same routine analysis of his patient's mental status that is commonly given to the alimentary, circulatory, excretory, neuromuscular and other function' [53].

As it happened in other fields of clinical medicine, a conceptual shift from a merely biomedical approach to a psychosomatic consideration of the person and his/her quality of life appears to be necessary for improving therapeutic effectiveness in endocrine disorders [54, 55].

References

1 Weitzner MA, Sonino N, Knutzen R (eds): Emotional Aspects of Pituitary Disease. Basel, Karger, 1998.
2 Sonino N, Fava GA: Psychological aspects of endocrine disease. Clin Endocrinol 1998;49:1–7.
3 Sobrinho LG: Psychopathology in endocrine disorders. Psychother Psychosom 2004;73:65–67.
4 Sonino N, Navarrini C, Ruini C, Ottolini F, Paoletta A, Fallo F, Boscaro M, Fava GA: Persistent psychological distress in patients treated for endocrine disease. Psychother Psychosom 2004;73:78–83.
5 Fava GA, Sonino N: The clinical domains of psychosomatic medicine. J Clin Psychiatry 2005;66: 849–855.
6 Vingerhoets AJJM, Assies J: Psychoneuroendocrinology of stress and emotions. Psychother Psychosom 1991;55:69–75.
7 Biondi M, Picardi A: Psychological stress and neuroendocrine function in humans: the last two decades of research. Psychother Psychosom 1999;68:114–150.
8 Paykel ES: The Interview for Recent Life events. Psychol Med 1997;27:301–310.

9 Sonino N, Fava GA, Boscaro M : A role for life events in the pathogenesis of Cushing's disease. Clin Endocrinol 1993;38:261–264.
10 Krieger DT: Pathophysiology of Cushing's disease. Endocr Rev 1983;4:22–43.
11 Sonino N, Girelli ME, Boscaro M, Fallo F, Busnardo B, Fava GA: Life events in the pathogenesis of Graves' disease. A controlled study. Acta Endocrinol 1993;128:293–296.
12 Winsa B, Adami HO, Bergstrom R, Gamstedt A, Dahlberg PA, Adamson U, Jansson R, Karlsson A: Stressful life events and Graves' disease. Lancet 1991;338:1475–1479.
13 Kung AWC: Life events, daily stresses and coping in patients with Graves' disease. Clin Endocrinol 1995;42:303–308.
14 Radosavljevic VR, Jakovic SM, Marinkovic JM: Stressful life events in the pathogenesis of Graves' disease. Eur J Endocrinol 1996;134:699–701.
15 Chrousos GP, Gold PW: The concepts of stress and stress system disorders. JAMA 1992;267: 1244–1252.
16 Sonino N, Navarrini C, Ruini C, Fallo F, Boscaro M, Fava GA: Life events in the pathogenesis of hyperprolactinemia. Eur J Endocrinol 2004;151:61–65.
17 Nunes MCP, Sobrinho L, Calhaz-Jorge C, Santes MA, Mauricio JC, Sousa MFF: Psychosomatic factors in patients with hyperprolactinemia and/or galactorrhea. Obstet Gynecol 1980;55: 591–595.
18 McEwen BS, Stellar E: Stress and the individual. Arch Intern Med 1993;153:2093–2101.
19 McEwen BS: Protective and damaging effects of stress mediators. N Engl J Med 1998;338: 171–179.
20 Pasquali R: The biological balance between psychological well-being and distress. Psychother Psychosom 2006;75:69–71.
21 Ryff CD, Love GL, Urry HL, Muller D, Rosenkranz MA, Friedmann EM, Davidson RJ, Singer B: Psychological well-being and ill-being. Psychother Psychosom 2006;75:85–95.
22 Sonino N, Fava GA: A simple instrument for assessing stress in clinical practice. Postgrad Med J 1998;74:408–410.
23 Sonino N, Ruini C, Navarrini C, Ottolini F, Sirri L, Paoletta A, Fallo F, Boscaro M, Fava GA: Psychosocial impairment in patients treated for pituitary disease. A controlled study. Clin Endocrinol (in press).
24 Fava GA, Freyberger HJ, Bech P, Christodoulou G, Sensky T, Theorell T, Wise TN: Diagnostic criteria for use in psychosomatic research. Psychother Psychosom 1995;63:1–8.
25 Fava GA, Morphy MA, Sonino N: Affective prodromes of medical illness. Psychother Psychosom 1994;62:141–145.
26 Fava GA, Sonino N: Depression associated with medical illness. CNS Drugs 1996;5:175–189.
27 Sonino N, Fava GA: Psychiatric disorders associated with Cushing's syndrome. CNS Drugs 2001;15:361–373.
28 Sonino N, Zielezny M, Fava GA, Fallo F, Boscaro M: Risk factors and long-term outcome in pituitary-dependent Cushing's disease. J Clin Endocrinol Metab 1996;81:2647–2652.
29 Josephson AM, Mackenzie TB: Thyroid induced mania in hypothyroid patients. Br J Psychiatry 1980;137:222–228.
30 Matsubayashi S, Tamai H, Matsumoto Y, Tamagana K, Mukuta T, Morita T, Kibio C: Graves' disease after the onset of panic disorder. Psychother Psychosom 1996;65:277–280.
31 Starkman MN, Zelnik TC, Nesse RM, Cameron OG: Anxiety in patients with pheochromocytoma. Arch Intern Med 1985;145:248–252.
32 Sonino N, Fallo F, Fava GA: Psychological aspects of primary aldosteronism. Psychother Psychosom 2006;75:327–330.
33 Stern RA, Robinson B, Thorner AR, Arruda JE, Prohaska ML, Prange AJ: A survey study of neuropsychiatric complaints in patients with Graves' disease. J Neuropsychiatry Clin Neurosci 1996;8:181–185.
34 Fava GA, Fava M, Kellner R, Serafini E, Mastrogiacomo I: Depression, hostility and anxiety in hyperprolactinemic amenorrhea. Psychother Psychosom 1981;6:122–128.
35 Kellner R, Buckman MT, Fava GA, Pathak D: Hyperprolactinemia, distress, and hostility. Am J Psychiatry 1984;141:759–763.
36 Keller SK, Neuhaus-Theil A, Quabbe HJ : Psychological correlates of prolactin secretion. Acta Endocrinol 1985;108:118–119.

37 Reavley S, Fisher AD, Owen D, Creed FH, Davis JRE: Psychological distress in patients with hyperprolactinemia. Clin Endocrinol 1997;47:343–348.
38 Buckman MT, Kellner R: Reduction of distress in hyperprolactinemia with bromocriptine. Am J Psychiatry 1985;142:242–244.
39 Mangelli L, Fava GA, Grassi L, Ottolini F, Paolini S, Porcelli P, Rafanelli C, Rigatelli M, Sonino N: Irritable mood in Italian patients with medical disease. J Nerv Ment Dis 2006;194:226–228.
40 Schmale AH, Engel GL: The giving up-given up complex illustrated on film. Arch Gen Psychiatry 1967;17:135–145.
41 Mangelli L, Fava GA, Grandi S, Grassi L, Ottolini F, Porcelli P, Rafanelli C, Rigatelli M, Sonino N: Assessing demoralization and depression in the setting of medical disease. J Clin Psychiatry 2005;66:391–394.
42 Lipowski ZJ: Somatization. Am J Psychiatry 1987;47:160–167.
43 Lipowski ZJ: Psychosocial aspects of disease. Ann Intern Med 1969;71:1197–1206.
44 Fava GA : The concept of psychosomatic disorder. Psychother Psychosom 1992;58:1–12.
45 Furman K, Ezzat S: Psychological features of acromegaly. Psychother Psychosom 1998;57: 147–153.
46 Burman P, Deijen JB: Quality of life and cognitive functions in patients with pituitary insufficiency. Psychother Psychosom 1998;67:154–167.
47 Uhde TW: Anxiety and growth disturbance: is there a connection? J Clin Psychiatry 1994;55 (suppl 6):17–27.
48 Wallymahmed ME, Baker GA, Humphris G, Dewey M, MacFarlane IA: The development, reliability and validity of a disease specific quality of life model for adults with growth hormone deficiency. Clin Endocrinol 1996;44:403–411.
49 McGauley G: Growth hormone treatment, brain neurotransmitters and thyroxine. Clin Endocrinol 1996;44:325–326.
50 Sonino N, Fava GA, Belluardo P, Girelli ME, Boscaro M: Course of depression in Cushing's syndrome: response to treatment and comparison with Graves' disease. Horm Res 1993;39:202–206.
51 Emanuele MA, Brooks MH, Gordon DL, Braithwaite SS: Agoraphobia and hyperthyroidism. Am J Med 1989;86:484–486.
52 Riedel M, Wiese A, Schurmeyer TH, Brabant G: Quality of life in patients with Addison's disease: effects of different cortisol replacement modes. Exp Clin Endocrinol 1993;101:106–111.
53 Cushing H: Psychic disturbances associated with disorders of the ductless glands. Am J Insanity 1913;69:965–990.
54 Fava GA, Sonino N, Morphy MA: Psychosomatic view of endocrine disorders. Psychother Psychosom 1993;59:20–33.
55 Boswell EB, Anfinson TJ, Nemeroff CB: Depression associated with endocrine disorders; in Robertson MM, Katona CLE (eds): Depression and Physical Illness. New York, Wiley, 1997, pp 255–292.

Nicoletta Sonino, MD
Department of Statistical Sciences, University of Padova
Via Battisti 241
IT–35121 Padova (Italy)
Tel. +39 049 827 4189, Fax +39 049 827 4170, E-Mail nicoletta.sonino@unipd.it

Porcelli P, Sonino N (eds): Psychological Factors Affecting Medical Conditions. A New Classification for DSM-V. Adv Psychosom Med. Basel, Karger, 2007, vol 28, pp 34–56

Psychological Factors Affecting Functional Gastrointestinal Disorders

Piero Porcelli[a], *Orlando Todarello*[b]

[a]Psychosomatic Unit, IRCCS De Bellis Hospital, Castellana Grotte, and [b]Department of Psychiatry, University of Bari, Bari, Italy

Abstract

Functional gastrointestinal disorders are a variable combination of chronic or recurrent medically unexplained gastrointestinal symptoms. They can be conceptualized within the biopsychosocial model of illness as a dysregulation of the brain-gut axis and its relationships with psychosocial variables (psychopathology, health care seeking, life events, somatosensory amplification). Psychopathology may be undetected with the standard psychiatric criteria, particularly at a subclinical level. Using the new classification of the Diagnostic Criteria for Psychosomatic Research (DCPR) for assessing psychosocial components of somatic illnesses, psychosomatic syndromes were found at a prevalence of 2.5 times greater than DSM-IV diagnoses. In particular, alexithymia, persistent somatization, functional somatic symptoms secondary to a psychiatric disorder, and demoralization were the most prevalent syndromes. Furthermore, psychosomatic severity (as measured with the presence of more than one DCPR conditions) strongly predicted the treatment outcome in patients with functional gastrointestinal disorders. In particular, alexithymia and persistent somatization were independent predictors of unimprovement (and health anxiety of improvement) after 6 months of treatment as usual, after controlling for gastrointestinal symptoms at baseline. DCPR may therefore be suggested as a reliable assessment instrument for psychological conditions that are relevant for psychosomatic practice and research settings but that are not included in the DSM-IV.

The functional gastrointestinal disorders (FGID) are broadly defined as a variable combination of chronic or recurrent gastrointestinal (GI) symptoms that are not explained by structural or biochemical abnormalities. The current consensus definition and criteria (the 'Rome III criteria') characterize FGID in terms of multiple physiological determinants that variously contribute to a set of syndromes involving the whole GI tract, from the esophagus to the anus [1].

Table 1. Diagnostic Rome III criteria for FD

1. One or more of the following symptoms must be present for the last 3 months, with onset at least 6 months before diagnosis:
   a. Bothersome postprandial fullness (occurring after ordinary-sized meals, at least several times per week)
   b. Early satiation (preventing finishing a regular meal, at least several times per week)
   c. Epigastric pain (localized to the epigastrium of at least moderate severity at least once per week, intermittent, not generalized or localized to other abdominal or chest regions, not relieved by defecation or passage of flatus)
   d. Epigastric burning (same characteristics of pain, without a retrosternal component)
2. No evidence of structural disease (including at upper endoscopy) that is likely to explain the symptoms

Table 2. Diagnostic Rome III criteria for IBS

Recurrent abdominal pain or discomfort at least 3 days per month in the last 3 months, with onset at least 6 months before diagnosis, associated with 2 or more of the following:
1. Improvement with defecation
2. Onset associated with a change in frequency of stools
3. Onset associated with a change in form of stool

Subtyping IBS by predominant stool pattern:
- Constipation (IBS-C): Hard or lumpy stools ≥25% and loose or watery stools <25% of bowel movements
- Diarrhea (IBS-D): Loose or watery stools ≥25% and hard or lumpy stool <25% of bowel movements
- Mixed IBS: Hard or lumpy stools ≥25% and loose or watery stools ≥25% of bowel movements
- Unspecified IBS: Insufficient abnormality of stools meeting criteria for the above

Functional dyspepsia (FD) and irritable bowel syndrome (IBS) are among the most common forms of FGID (tables 1 and 2).

Although criteria define syndromes for each different segment of the GI tract, symptoms often overlap and fluctuate over time, but syndromes are considered relatively stable because the disappearance of symptoms in some individuals is balanced by similar rates of new onsets. It has been estimated that the prevalence of FGID is between 10 and 20% in the general population but as high as 40–50% in clinical practice, gastroenterology settings, and primary care. The economic impact of IBS is enormous. High direct costs are due to frequent consultations, pointless tests, inappropriate management, and even unnecessary surgery while indirect costs are mainly due to work or school absenteeism [1–4].

Although the pathophysiology of FGID is not fully understood, there is accumulating evidence that symptom formation involves an interaction among multiple factors that vary in importance from one patient to another. These factors include motility disturbances, altered thresholds of pain and other sensory input from the gut, GI inflammation and infection, psychological distress, and personality disturbances [5, 6]. The aim of this work was to review published data on psychological factors affecting symptom presentation and treatment outcome in FGID patients with the Diagnostic Criteria for Psychosomatic Research (DCPR) [7].

Biopsychosocial Model and Functional Gastrointestinal Disorders

The multidisciplinary nature of the FGID challenges the basic assumption of the biomedical model of Western medicine, according to which diseases are caused by identifiable abnormalities in the structure and function of organs and tissues that in turn have a causal and linear relationship to the individual's perception of ill health. However this kind of correlation between disease and subjective perception of symptom does not seem to fit with FGID symptoms. Some physicians may feel frustration when making a diagnosis of FGID because they are trained to seek pathology and are not at ease with somatic symptoms at the interface between the medical and the psychological fences of the clinical field, and therefore they tend to see FGID as a disease with unknown medical causes [8]. On the other hand, psychiatric classification of functional somatic disorders is poorly adequate and may lead to the unjustified attribution of psychological problems that patients do not have, exaggeration of psychological problems that they do have, and the neglect of any physical problems that are present [9].

Conversely, in the biopsychosocial model [10] illness is viewed as a multifactorial entity resulting from interaction of systems at cellular, tissue, organism, interpersonal and environmental levels. Psychosocial stress may therefore exacerbate GI symptoms and modify the experience of illness and illness behavior such as health care seeking. In turn, chronic GI disorders may have psychosocial consequences on one's general well-being and daily functioning [11]. Even if symptoms may have a more prominent physiological or psychological basis, no single physiological or psychological cause is responsible for symptoms of FGID. Rather, FGID can be conceived as a group of biopsychosocial disorders resulting from interaction of multiple systems such as the nervous system, psychological factors, altered intestinal motility, and increased sensitivity [12]. In such interacting systems, events do not occur in isolation. For example, activated immunocompetent cells in the intestinal mucosa have been found to be increased in patients with IBS [13]. Psychosocial stressors may modulate the immune response of the gut to infectious agents, and in turn, gut-directed physiological stressors may modulate the responsiveness of the central nervous system. Altered outputs of central stress circuits, such as the hypothalamus-pituitary-adrenal axis and the sympathetic arousal of the autonomous nervous system, may alter the gut immune system and increase intestinal permeability, thereby increasing susceptibility to inflammatory agents in the gut lumen [14]. The vulnerability to psychological problems or the development of gut dysfunction may be determined by the alteration of the brain-gut axis and/or stressful events or genetic and environmental (from major loss to history of abuse to exposure to infections) factors in early life [12].

In summary, as claimed by Drossman [15], 'it is no longer rational to try to discriminate whether physiological or psychologic factors produce pain or other bowel symptoms, dysmotility, or inflammation. Instead, [FGID] seem to be understood in terms of dysregulation of brain-gut function, and the task is to determine the degree to which each is operative and remediable' (p. 4).

Psychiatric Comorbidity of Functional Gastrointestinal Disorders

The comorbidity of psychiatric disorders with FGID is well established in studies using reliable diagnostic instruments and documented in clinical practice [5, 6]. Although no single psychiatric disorder has been linked to FGID, the prevalence of psychiatric diagnoses, most frequently mood and anxiety disorders, ranges between 40 and 100%, depending on the population, settings, and diagnostic criteria [16, 17]. Also, although less information is available for the inverse association, complaints of functional bowel symptoms (altered bowel habit, abdominal discomfort, bloating) have been found in 30–70% of patients with psychiatric disorders [18, 19]. We were able to replicate these findings in patients recruited in a GI outpatient facility and a psychiatric outpatient clinic [20]. Thirty-eight of 58 (65.5%) patients with FGID had also a DSM-IV diagnosis and 25 of 52 (48%) psychiatric patients fulfilled the Rome criteria for FGID. While 88% of psychiatric patients with GI syndromes had a mood or anxiety disorders, GI patients with psychiatric comorbidity had anxiety, mood, somatoform, and adjustment disorders, at a rate of almost 25% for each diagnosis.

The high rate of co-occurrence of FGID and psychopathology is generally not interpreted as if the two classes of disorders were directly and/or causally linked. Psychiatric disturbances might however be conceptualized as one of the necessary but not sufficient substrates for the occurrence of FGID, while the reverse is not necessarily found. Furthermore, FGID patients referred to tertiary care are more psychologically disturbed that those referred to primary care [21], so that the close association between FGID and psychopathology should not be regarded as a characteristic of the illness per se but as more strictly related to the patient's health care seeking behavior [22]. However, there is another possible explanation, namely that the official diagnostic criteria included in the DSM-IV are limited and less effective when applied to medical patients, and therefore should be integrated with different criteria for psychological syndromes affecting these clinical conditions.

Psychosocial Mediators in Functional Gastrointestinal Disorders

Even though symptoms of FGID wax and wane, a subgroup of patients might be vulnerable to experience prolonged periods of symptoms or to report medically unexplained symptoms in different body sites ('serial' or 'chronic somatizers') [23]. Using different statistical methods, two independent studies on patients with a variety of functional somatic syndromes found that a general somatization latent factor accounted for up to 69% of the total variances of symptoms, and that IBS symptom clustering was a second-order variable distinct from other functional non-GI disorders [24, 25]. A recent meta-analysis found that IBS as well as other medically unexplained syndromes were related to (but not fully dependent on) depression and anxiety [26]. In addition, IBS symptoms may change their clinical manifestation, as shown by patients with past eating disorders who later developed functional FGID [27] and cholecystectomized patients with persistent functional GI symptoms 1 year after surgery [28].

Some of the suggested psychological constructs as probable mediating factors in the experience, reporting, and persistence of FGID will be briefly discussed here.

Health Care Seeking Behavior

Several epidemiological studies suggest that people with IBS symptoms who do not consult a physician are psychologically similar to asymptomatic population. In contrast, subjects with IBS who seek health care have more anxiety, depression, health anxiety, hypochondriacal concerns and are less likely to see a link between stress and their symptoms. The prevalence of these psychological disturbances is greater in tertiary care settings [29, 30]. A recent longitudinal study has investigated the association between change of psychological and bowel symptoms over a 1-year period in a community sample [2]. Although not associated with symptom change over time, psychological distress predicted the persistence of GI symptoms and health care seeking. In particular, greater anxiety or worry about visceral pain in the preceding weeks was an independent predictor of frequent medical visits for severely perceived bowel symptoms.

These data suggest that psychological symptoms are not associated with the IBS per se but with the decision to consult a physician, possibly a specialist, and therefore with health care seeking. FGID consulters were found to have higher scores on somatization, emotionality, quality of life, health rating, and social support than general population. Furthermore, repression and disease conviction were strong and independent predictors of the frequency of physician consultations, along with illness variables such as severity and duration of symptoms [31].

Sexual and Physical Abuse

In 1990s, several studies found a higher prevalence of self-reported sexual and physical abuse in FGID patients (up to 67% in the US and 32% in Europe) [32, 33]. These data suggest that sexual abuse contributes to the development of FGID, perhaps through downregulation of visceral sensitivity threshold, guilt, maladaptive adjustment, and hypervigilance to illness complaints in early life [1]. However, numerous methodological problems have been highlighted in such research. In a population-based survey, abuse was associated with both neuroticism and IBS, but abuse was not associated with IBS after controlling for neuroticism and psychological morbidity [34]. The link between abuse and IBS may therefore be mediated by neuroticism, a personality trait characterized by exaggerated responsivity to physiological changes. In fact, childhood abuse has been found to be associated with higher levels of current psychological distress, irrespective of having IBS, idiopathic constipation, or Crohn's disease [35].

It is likely that sexual abuse is not a cause of FGID. Rather, a more conservative explanation is that abuse is a strong stressful experience with consequences that may last all life long, predisposing individuals to psychological and somatic vulnerability. Consistently with Lipowski's [36] somatization construct, the consequences of abuse may be better conceived as associated to a tendency to communicate psychological distress through somatic symptoms, thus contributing to symptom maintenance and health care seeking. In fact, longitudinal data have shown chronic highly threatening stressors significantly and unequivocally predicted IBS symptom intensity and clinical outcome, independent of other confounders, and not the reverse [37].

Somatosensory Amplification

One of the important clinical features of FGID is pain, namely a subjective dimension of health perception mostly influenced by possible dysregulation of the bidirectional brain-gut axis. A large amount of studies have consistently found lower pain threshold perception during rectal distension, or 'visceral hyperalgesia', in IBS patients compared to healthy subjects [38]. Stress, anxiety, selective attention, or recall of aversive memories can enhance perception of painful stimuli [39, 40] whereas distraction and relaxation can decrease perceptual sensitivity [41].

Visceral hyperalgesia may be conceived as the physiologic counterpart of the psychological construct of 'somatosensory amplification', that is an amplifying perceptual style entailing a hypervigilance or heightened attentional focus on bodily sensations, a tendency to select out and attend to certain bodily sensations, and a propensity for responding to them with affect and cognitions that make them more disturbing and intense [42]. It is related to the cognitive schemata that individuals use to interpret physical sensations, to label them as signs of poor health, and to report them to the physician as evidence of clinical symptoms. Cognitive attribution of physical symptoms to somatic rather than psychological causes (somatic attributional style) is greater in patients with chronic functional medical disorders than psychiatric illness [43].

Cognitive schemas, as catastrophizing and social desirability, may contribute to somatosensory amplification and play a mediating role between perception, psychopathology and behavior. Catastrophizing, the tendency to focus on and exaggerate the threat value of painful stimuli, has been widely studied in chronic pain patients and was found to partly mediate the effect between depression and pain in IBS patients. Patients with IBS who experience higher levels of depression engage in more catastrophic thinking, and partly through this thinking style experience more intense pain and greater activity limitations due to pain (i.e. pain severity). Also, IBS patients showed higher scores on social desirability [44]. They may inappropriately and repeatedly subject themselves to unnecessary and even harmful medical procedures in search of treatment for an illness with an organic cause. In another words, individuals may pay attention to their GI sensations if they are afraid they may have a disease and, in turn, becoming increasingly aware of their GI sensations may reinforce their belief.

DCPR Diagnoses in Functional Gastrointestinal Disorders

Prevalence of DCPR Syndromes in Functional Gastrointestinal Disorders

Based on population studies, there is a general consensus that psychological factors do not affect FGID per se. Rather, psychological abnormalities characterize a small proportion of 20–30% of FGID people under treatment (consulters or patients) who are psychologically different from people who have FGID symptoms but who do not refer to physicians (nonconsulters or nonpatients). A German study has found, in a representative sample of 2,201 subjects from general population, that 288 individuals (13.1%) met the criteria for FGID and about one half of whom had seen a physician because of their GI symptoms in the previous year (corresponding to 6.7% of the total sample) [31]. Three clusters of variables accounted for 40% of the variance in the frequency of medical consultations: illness variables (acute episodes, symptom severity, and health rating), psychological factors (somatization, depression, emotionality, and life events), and cognitive somatic rather than psychological attribution of their symptoms. In a recent study, we compared FGID patients with comorbid DSM-IV psychopathology referred to a gastroenterology department with psychiatric outpatients who also met the Rome criteria for FGID who were seen in a psychiatric setting [20]. FGID patients with psychiatric disorders were more alexithymic and had less psychopathology than psychiatric patients with FGID, but GI symptoms were not significantly different. Therefore, higher level of alexithymia seems to characterize referral to a medical care setting, whereas more severe psychopathology referral to psychiatric care, after controlling for GI symptoms. Furthermore, FGID patients referred to tertiary care were found to have higher abnormal illness behavior, psychosocial disturbances, health care seeking behavior, psychiatric diagnoses, activity disruption, and less physiological correlates for their symptoms than FGID patients referred to primary care [1]. If these findings are seen from a psychosomatic perspective, the situation can be reframed by claiming that those patients show a somatization process, conceived with Lipowski [36] as the results of both the tendency to experience psychological distress in the form of physical symptoms *and* to seek medical help for them.

In a series of 190 consecutive patients (64% of whom were women, aged on average 37 years) with FGID referred to a hospital-based, tertiary care center, psychological disturbances were evaluated with DSM-IV and DCPR. Eighty-three patients (44%) fulfilled the criteria for FD, 38 (20%) for IBS, 40 (21%) for both FD and IBS, and 29 (15%) for functional abdominal pain. A quarter of the patients (n = 48) received no DSM-IV diagnosis. In the remaining 142 patients, somatoform disorders, as expected, were the most frequent diagnostic category (n = 56; 29%), followed by adjustment disorders (n = 42; 22%) and mood disorders (n = 39; 20%); 43 patients (23%) had a DSM-IV diagnosis of axis II personality disorder.

Table 3 shows the prevalence of DCPR syndromes evaluated with the structural interview for DCPR [45]. Only 17 patients (9%) received no DCPR diagnosis. In the remaining 173 patients, alexithymia (n = 90; 47%), persistent somatization (n = 64; 34%), functional somatic symptoms secondary to a psychiatric disorder (n = 56; 29%), and demoralization (n = 43; 23%) were the most frequent diagnostic findings and accounted for almost three quarters of the diagnoses.

Table 3. Ranking order of DCPR syndromes in FGID

Rank	DCPR categories	n	%
1	Alexithymia	90	47.4
2	Persistent somatization	64	33.7
3	FSS	56	29.5
4	Demoralization	43	22.6
5	Disease phobia	23	12.1
6	Health anxiety	22	11.6
7	Irritable mood	20	10.5
8	Type A behavior	16	8.4
9	Conversion symptoms	9	4.7
10	Illness denial	7	3.7
11	Thanatophobia	3	1.6
12	Anniversary reaction	1	0.5

FSS = Functional somatic symptoms secondary to a psychiatric disorder.

Table 4 shows the proportions of patients with DSM-IV diagnoses overlapping to DCPR syndromes (below the diagonal) and vice versa (above the diagonal). Only the most frequent diagnostic categories (with both diagnostic criteria) are reported.

Mood disorders were frequently associated with alexithymia (67%) and functional somatic symptoms secondary to a psychiatric disorder (56%). Somatoform disorders were more related to alexithymia (48%) than persistent somatization (34%). The overlaps of patients with DCPR syndromes who also received DSM-IV diagnoses were lower compared to the previous associations. Only 9 (5%) of the patients received neither a DCPR nor a DSM diagnosis.

There were considerable overlaps between the DCPR diagnoses of alexithymia and persistent somatization. Interestingly, the overlap between persistent somatization and functional somatic symptoms secondary to a psychiatric diagnosis was very low (8%). There were fewer patients with no DCPR diagnosis (n = 17; 9%) than with no DSM-IV diagnoses (n = 48; 25%), more patients with one DSM-IV diagnosis (n = 110; 58%) than with one DCPR diagnosis (n = 47; 25%), and more patients with two or more DCPR diagnoses (n = 122; 64%) than with multiple DSM-IV diagnoses (n = 32; 17%). Only 9 (19%) of the 48 patients who received no DSM diagnosis were not identified by DCPR. Alexithymia, functional somatic symptoms secondary to a psychiatric disorder, demoralization and persistent somatization were the most frequent DCPR diagnostic findings also in the remaining 39 patients.

Table 4. Overlap rates of DCPR syndromes to DSM-IV diagnoses (below the diagonal) and DSM-IV diagnoses to DCPR syndromes (above the diagonal)

	Mood disorders (n = 39)	Somatoform disorders (n = 56)	Adjustment disorders (n = 42)	Anxiety disorders (n = 28)
Alexithymia	28.9	30.0	14.4	12.2
(n = 90)	66.7	48.2	30.9	39.3
Persistent	26.5	29.7	12.5	15.6
somatization (n = 64)	43.6	33.9	19.0	35.7
FSS	39.3	16.1	26.2	17.8
(n = 56)	56.4	16.1	26.2	35.7
Demoralization	30.2	20.9	14.4	4.6
(n = 43)	33.3	16.1	30.9	7.1

These findings indicate that DCPR may be viewed as encompassing psychosomatic and subclinical symptomatology, and therefore can be used jointly with the DSM-IV for assessing psychiatric disorders. Most patients who were identified by the DCPR as showing one or more psychological conditions were not detected by the psychopathology criteria of the DSM-IV. In particular, the ratio of the number of DSM-IV to DCPR categories in our sample was 1 to 2.5. In particular, a quarter of patients did not fulfill diagnostic criteria for any DSM-IV disorder, while less than 10% did not receive any DCPR diagnosis; 17% of patients fulfilled criteria for at least one DCPR category but no DSM-IV disorder, while less than 4% of patients received at least one DSM-IV category but no DCPR diagnosis. Therefore, the number of DCPR/not-DSM patients was 4.7 times higher than that of DSM/not-DCPR patients.

About half of patients had alexithymia, more than one third persistent somatization, and about one quarter demoralization. Although frequent in our as well as other clinical samples, none of these psychosomatic conditions is included in the DSM-IV. This result is particularly impressive if one considers that the prevalence of the DSM-IV categories of somatoform and adjustment disorders in our sample was of 29 and 22%, respectively. The difference in the two classification systems is particularly evident when similar constructs are compared, i.e. functional secondary somatic symptoms and axis I disorders, and demoralization and mood disorders.

One of the cardinal rules of the DSM-IV is the hierarchical principle according to which somatic symptoms should not be secondary to other psychiatric disorders which have been often judged to be prominent over the somatoform symptoms. Medically unexplained symptoms are therefore placed at the same level as other axis I syndromes [46]. Many somatoform syndromes are thus underdiagnosed because the clinician assumes that another axis I disorder (mostly within the anxiety and depression spectrum) is prominent over the somatic symptoms. The DCPR criteria for 'functional somatic symptoms secondary to a psychiatric disorder' posit that a psychiatric disorder precedes the onset of symptoms of autonomic arousal or functional medical disorder. Therefore, patients may receive such DCPR diagnosis in the presence of an axis I disorder but also their symptoms might be associated with other psychosomatic factors, even if anxiety or depression might be thought to be clinically evident. As a result, it is not surprising that in more than half of our cases of mood and anxiety disorders, FGID were not judged to be secondary to psychopathology.

The DCPR criteria for demoralization include a prolonged feeling state, preceding the onset or the exacerbation of a medical condition, characterized by the individual sense of failure to meet one's own or others' expectations or inability to cope with pressing problems. Several clinical manifestations of demoralization may overlap with symptoms of mood disorder. In our sample, 23% of patients received a DCPR diagnosis of demoralization and 20% a DSM-IV diagnosis of mood disorder, although about only 30% of patients were classified with both. This is consistent with the results from a large study (n = 807) in which DCPR-related demoralization was found in 30% of patients, DSM-IV major depression in 17% of patients, although only 30–50% of them received both diagnoses [47]. Also, demoralization was found in 25% of 556 patients attending secondary health care clinics [48] and was the first-order dimension in a latent trait analysis of a wide range of symptoms in a large group of patients referred to consultation-liaison psychiatry [49]. Furthermore, demoralization was found in the identical proportion of 20% in both FGID groups who improved and not improved after treatment [50]. The DCPR category of demoralization is conceptually close to the 'giving-up syndrome complex', as a facilitating factor for the onset of disease to which the individual is predisposed [51], and is phenomenologically different from major depression [52]. Both demoralized and depressed patients experience a lack of motivation and drive, which influences their ability to interact in daily life. In the depressed patients, this inhibition is due to a primary reduction in motivation and drive and not to their incapacity to act, whereas in the demoralized persons, motivation and drive are usually intact but the lack of confidence and the feeling of helplessness inhibit their initiative [53]. The fact that demoralization was frequent in FGID patients, regardless of their symptom change after treatment, suggests that it may be a chronic feeling state that is not alleviated by improvement or persistence of somatic symptoms, as mood condition has often been found in the medically ill [54], and that probably needs specific psychological treatment.

DCPR Predictors of Treatment Outcome in Functional Gastrointestinal Disorders

The clinical utility of a diagnostic instrument can be thought of as a function of the degree and the amount of influence that the instrument has on multiple decisions and outcomes in clinical practice [55]. Concepts included in the construct of clinical utility are therefore related not only to classification but also to monitoring and predicting symptom change and treatment outcome [56]. We therefore evaluated the clinical utility of the DCPR classification, particularly the ability to predict treatment outcome in FGID patients [50].

One hundred and five patients of the 190 recruited in the previous study were evaluated at baseline and after 6 months of treatment as usual (TAU) with the structured interview for the DCPR and the Gastrointestinal Symptom Rating Scale (GSRS) [57], a rating scale including 15 GI symptoms rated on a 7-point Likert scale ranging from 0 (no symptoms) to 3 (pronounced symptoms), including half points (higher score indicate more severe symptoms). The GSRS total score was used to categorize patients into improved and unimproved outcome groups. Patients had to satisfy two criteria to be included in the improved group. The first criterion was determined by the change in overall GI symptoms, expressed as the proportion of change from baseline to follow-up (baseline minus follow-up GSRS total score divided by the GSRS total score at baseline). The mean GSRS total score change was 50.8%, and the median score change was 71.4%. Since a positive change in more than two thirds could be reasonably considered as a good clinical improvement of symptoms, we considered improved those patients who showed 67.1% (median value) of symptom change. By itself, however, this criterion is not sufficient to define a responder because overall symptoms at baseline may vary greatly among patients. The second criterion was therefore a low level of symptoms at follow-up. The mean GSRS total score at follow-up was 5.8 (SD = 6.0) and the median was 3 (range: 0–25; a higher score represents higher level of symptoms). We considered improved those patients who obtained a GSRS total score of ≤3 at follow-up (median score). Thus, using both criteria, the improved group included 65 patients with at least 71% of GSRS total score change from baseline to follow-up, and a GSRS total score of ≤3 at follow-up while the unimproved group was formed by 40 patients. TAU was delivered case by case with combination forms of GI medications (usually antisecretory, prokinetic and antispasmodic drugs), diet modifications (usually including high fiber intake), psychotropic medications (usually anxiolytic and antidepressant drugs, in low doses), psychological counseling, and/or brief psychotherapy. The two outcome-related groups were not different in sociodemographic variables and the kind of delivered treatment, while the unimproved group was significantly more severely symptomatic at baseline.

Table 5. DCPR syndromes in improved and unimproved FGID groups at baseline

	Improved patients n (%)	Unimproved patients n (%)	χ^2
Alexithymia	15 (23.1)	33 (82.2)	35.23***
Persistent somatization	7 (10.8)	29 (72.5)	41.88***
Health anxiety	14 (21.5)	1 (2.5)	7.33**
Disease phobia	5 (7.7)	9 (22.5)	4.70*
FSS	18 (27.7)	7 (17.5)	1.42
Irritable mood	5 (7.7)	6 (15.0)	1.41
Illness denial	3 (4.6)	0	1.90
Type A behavior	7 (10.8)	3 (7.5)	0.31
Conversion symptoms	3 (4.6)	1 (2.5)	0.30
Thanatophobia	1 (1.5)	0	0.62
Demoralization	13 (20.0)	8 (20.0)	0
Anniversary reaction	0	0	
DCPR = 0	15 (23.1)	0	9.94**
DCPR > 1	25 (38.5)	36 (90.0)	27.01***

*p < 0.05; **p < 0.01; ***p < 0.001.

Table 5 shows the frequency of DCPR diagnoses in the two outcome-related groups. The proportion of patients diagnosed with alexithymia, persistent somatization and, to a much minor extent, disease phobia was significantly higher in the unimproved (82, 72, and 22%, respectively) than in the improved group (23, 11, and 8%, respectively). Conversely, the proportion of patients with health anxiety was significantly increased in the improved (21%) compared to the unimproved group (2%). Of interest, the same high proportion of patients with demoralization was found in both groups (20%). Patients were also divided into three groups on the basis of the number of DCPR diagnoses, i.e. patients without any DCPR diagnosis (DCPR = 0), with one DCPR diagnosis (DCPR = 1), and with multiple DCPR diagnoses (DCPR > 1). All unimproved patients obtained at least one DCPR, while 23% improved patients had no DCPR diagnosis. Also, a significantly higher percentage of unimproved patients had multiple DCPR diagnoses (90%) compared to improved patients (38%).

To investigate which variables predicted best treatment outcome, two regression models were performed (table 6). In the first model (table 6, upper section), all the 12 DCPR diagnoses and the GSRS total score at baseline were considered as predictors. The final model resulting from the backward stepwise procedure showed that alexithymia and persistent somatization significantly

Table 6. DCPR predictors of treatment outcome (logistic regression)

	β	SE	OR	95% CI
Alexithymia	2.49	0.62	12.07	3.57–40.74
Health anxiety	2.39	1.27	10.90	0.01–1.11
Persistent somatization	2.71	0.63	14.98	4.32–51.94
DCPR > 1	2.67	0.58	14.40	4.57–45.37
GSRS total	0.90	0.46	2.99	1.00–1.97

predicted unimprovement while health anxiety had a significant buffer effect on unimprovement. Of interest, GI symptom severity (GSRS total score) did not enter in the final regression model. The model accurately predicted 91% of the improved and 73% of the unimproved patients (overall correct classification rate = 84%). In the second model (table 6, lower section), DCPR severity and symptom severity were considered as predictors. Using DCPR severity, patients fell into three categories with no, one, and more than one DCPR diagnosis. Greater DCPR severity (DCPR > 1) and, although at a much lesser extent, greater symptom severity at baseline (GSRS total score) significantly predicted unimprovement. The accuracy prediction of this model was lower than in the first model, with 74% of the improved patients and 75% of the unimproved patients being correctly classified (overall correct classification rate = 74%).

These results showed that FGID patients who did not respond to TAU were all diagnosed with at least one DCPR category and were more likely to have multiple DCPR clusters (90%) than improved patients. The severity of psychosomatic disturbance (measured as presence of more than one DCPR syndrome) may constitute a useful clinical indicator for treatment planning of 'difficult patients', i.e. patients with severe symptoms of somatization or GI medically unexplained symptoms. In particular, three main DCPR categories were found to be strongly associated with the TAU outcomes in FGID patients, two (alexithymia and persistent somatization) with unimprovement and one (health anxiety) with improvement.

Alexithymia is a cluster of cognitive and affective characteristics including difficulty identifying and communicating feelings, trouble distinguishing between feelings and somatic sensations of emotional arousal, impoverished and restrictive imaginative life, and a concrete and reality-oriented thinking style. Furthermore, it is conceived as personality trait of individuals with higher vulnerability to suffer from somatic as well as psychopathological disorders of affect regulation [58]. Prevalence of alexithymia, assessed with the 20-item Toronto Alexithymia Scale (TAS-20) [58], ranged from 12% in North-American FD patients [59] to 43 and

66%, in Italian samples of IBS [60] and FGID patients [61], respectively. Furthermore, alexithymia was found to influence referral to medical versus psychiatric health care settings [20] of patients with comorbid psychiatric and FGID disorders. Finally, alexithymia is thought to be involved in the treatment outcome of somatic patients [62]. In a sample of FGID patients, alexithymia, assessed at baseline with the TAS-20, was able to predict the final recovery status of unimprovement after treatment, even after controlling for baseline GI and psychological symptoms [63]. The DCPR criteria for alexithymia include at least 3 of the following 6 characteristics: inability to use appropriate words to describe emotions, tendency to describe details instead of feelings, lack of a rich fantasy life, thought content associated more with external events rather than fantasy or emotions, unawareness of the common somatic reactions that accompany the experience of a variety of feelings, occasional but violent and often inappropriate outbursts of affective behavior. Two studies evaluated the diagnostic efficiency of the DCPR alexithymia category against the TAS in Japanese psychiatric outpatients [64] and Italian FGID patients [65] and found consistent figures of sensitivity (67.4 and 70.2%, respectively) and specificity (74.7 and 81.6%, respectively). In our study on treatment outcome, the DCPR alexithymia syndrome was highly frequent in the unimproved group (82%) and the first independent predictor of symptom unimprovement. There are several potential pathways by which alexithymia might influence symptom severity and treatment outcome for FGID patients. These include a limited ability of high alexithymia individuals to cope adaptively with stressful situations, which may contribute to high levels of psychological distress, and a possible sustained arousal of the physiological component of emotion response systems. In addition, high alexithymia individuals may be prone to functional somatic symptoms because of a tendency to amplify, focus on, and misinterpret the somatic sensations that accompany states of emotional arousal as well as other normal bodily sensations (somatosensory amplification) [58, 62, 66]. Consequently, patients with high alexithymia may experience more severe somatic symptoms and respond poorly to treatment because of the difficulty in cognitively processing emotional and somatic stimuli.

Persistent somatization was the second most frequent DCPR diagnosis in unimproved patients (72.5%) and independent predictor of unimprovement. The DCPR criteria for persistent somatization require that in the previous 6 months the subject had experienced significant somatic symptoms (e.g. aches, fatigue, dyspepsia, dizziness and tachycardia) without organic cause that caused repeated medical care and impaired the quality of life, and suffered from exaggerated side effects from medical therapy. The concept of persistent somatization derives from Kellner's [67] review of the medical literature. Kellner suggested that it may be clinically advantageous to conceptualize a somatizing patient as someone in whom psychological symptoms have clustered. In particular, he thought that the conception of persistent somatization as symptom clustering is justified by the clinical observations that people likely to get one medically unexplained symptom are more likely to subsequently get another medically unexplained symptom than those without a history of repeated unexplained symptoms. Other authors have used different labels to capture the characteristics of persistent symptoms in somatizing patients and therefore to overcome the too stringent criteria of the DSM-IV somatization disorder and the too broad DSM-IV criteria of undifferentiated somatoform disorder. Categories similar to DCPR persistent somatization are multisomatoform disorder [68], pure somatizers [69], or chronic somatizers [70]. The concept of persistent somatization is therefore related to psychological features theoretically consistent with lower probabilities of improvement after therapy, as individuals have a high dissatisfaction with their health, multiple and long-standing physical symptoms, a tendency to somatic amplification leading to increased symptom report, high disease conviction, and therefore a low ability to subjectively perceive symptom reduction with treatment [71].

Health anxiety was significantly more prevalent in improved (21.5%) than unimproved (2.5%) patients and also a significant independent predictor of improvement. Although they might seem similar, health anxiety and hypochondriasis are phenomenologically heterogeneous and characterize different subgroups of psychological features in subjects with overlapping symptom manifestations. The DCPR criteria for health anxiety require that the subject is highly concerned with health worries and fears for having a serious disease, as in the DSM-IV hypochondriasis, but this feeling state is of short duration (less than 6 months) and is easily reduced by appropriate medical explanations on the nature of the physical symptoms. Conversely, the DSM-IV criteria of hypochondriasis require a long-lasting, nondelusional worry or fear of having a serious disease that is based on misinterpretation of physical symptoms or sensations and not relieved by appropriate medical evaluation and reassurance that no illness is present. Therefore, while the doctor-patient relationship is less likely to change the individual beliefs of hypochondriacal patients, it may influence greatly, at least in the short-term, the emotional arousal that accompanies the patients' anxiety on their current symptoms. That might explain why somatic anxiety of hypochondriacal type is associated with poor health status, while health anxiety, as defined by DCPR, may alleviate the patients' concerns. In fact, having greater anxiety or worry about abdominal symptoms in the weeks preceding medical consultation and greater psychological distress were found to be important independent predictors of frequently seeking medical care for GI symptoms over time [2]. However, health anxiety may be also a psychological state fostering adaptation and recovery. For instance, health anxiety was high in women before thermography and mammography but significantly decreased after the communication of the negative result from the examination [72]. The improvement in FGID patients with health anxiety may be related to a placebo-like effect determined by the kind of therapy provided. The treatment format in our investigation consisted of different forms of therapy (including GI and psychotropic medications, diet modification, psychological counseling, and brief psychotherapy) that were combined in various ways on a case by case basis. Counseling was always provided to patients even though they were treated only with drugs, therefore involving those therapeutic ingredients that are thought to be part of the placebo response, such as regularly scheduled visits during the follow-up, education, reassurance and ongoing relationship [73, 74]. This therapeutic approach to FGID is quite usual in clinical practice [12]. Placebo response is frequent in FGID treatments at an average rate of 40% (range 16–71%) [30, 75]. A striking symptom improvement of 80% was reported in FD patients treated with placebo that was independent of changes in GI motility or gastric hypersensitivity to distension [76]. In agreement with the literature, our findings suggest that expectations of symptom relief from treatment, a more positive attitude towards health care providers, and a reduction in anxiety may constitute a powerful, unspecific therapeutic instrument in patients with health anxiety.

Conclusion

Using DSM-IV criteria in medical settings a basic question arises: whether patients who do not fulfill these criteria do not indeed present with psychological problems which may affect the medical symptoms and are worthy of clinical attention. The DCPR have been designed to answer to the need of clinicians in evaluating medical patients who are not detected by the DSM-IV criteria. Findings from studies using the DCPR in FGID patients referred to tertiary care suggest that the DCPR are able to detect psychological dimensions and/or subthreshold psychopathology which are not identified by the DSM-IV categories, particularly alexithymia, persistent somatization, and demoralization, and that DCPR categories are able to predict the treatment outcome, particularly alexithymia and persistent somatization are associated with unimprovement and health anxiety improvement after TAU (table 7).

The symptom formation in FGID involves a complex interaction among multiple factors that vary in importance from one patient to another. These factors include motility disturbances, altered thresholds of pain and other sensory input from the gut, GI inflammation and infection, psychological distress, and personality disturbances [6]. Personality traits and emotional states may not only induce effects on the physiology of the gut, but also influence how the symptoms of FGID are experienced and acted upon, and the outcome of treatment. The

53 Clarke DM, Kissane DW: Demoralization: its phenomenology and importance. Aust N Z J Psychiatry 2002;36:733–742.
54 von Ammon Cavanaugh: Depression in medically ill. Clinical issues in diagnostic assessment. Psychosomatics 1995;36:48–59.
55 Murphy KR, Davidshofer CO: Psychological Testing. Principles and Applications, ed 2. Englewood Cliffs, Prentice Hall, 1991.
56 Foster SL, Cone JD: Validity issues in clinical assessment. Psychol Assess 1995;7:248–260.
57 Svedlund J, Sjödin I, Dotevall G: GSRS. A clinical rating scale for gastrointestinal symptoms in patients with irritable bowel syndrome and peptic ulcer disease. Dig Dis Sci 1988;33:129–134.
58 Taylor GJ, Bagby RM, Parker JDA: Disorders of affect regulation. Alexithymia in medical and psychiatric illness. Cambridge, Cambridge University, 1997.
59 Jones MP, Schettler A, Olden K, Crowell MD: Alexithymia and somatosensory amplification in functional dyspepsia. Psychosomatics 2004;45:508–516.
60 Portincasa P, Moschetta A, Baldassarre G, Altomare DF, Palasciano G: Pan-enteric dysmotility, impaired quality of life and alexithymia in a large group of patients meeting Rome II criteria for irritable bowel syndrome. World J Gastroenterol 2003;9:2293–2299.
61 Porcelli P, Taylor GJ, Bagby RM, De Carne M: Alexithymia and functional gastrointestinal disorders. A comparison with inflammatory bowel disease. Psychother Psychosom 1999;68: 263–269.
62 Taylor GJ, Bagby RM: New trends in alexithymia research. Psychother Psychosom 2004;73: 68–77.
63 Porcelli P, Bagby RM, Taylor GJ, De Carne M, Leandro G, Todarello O: Alexithymia as a predictor of treatment in patients with functional gastrointestinal disorders. Psychosom Med 2003;65: 911–918.
64 Fukunishi I, Hosaka T, Aoki T, Azekawa T, Ota A, Miyaoka H: Criterion-related validity of diagnostic criteria for alexithymia in a general hospital psychiatric setting. Psychother Psychosom 1996;65:82–85.
65 Porcelli P, De Carne M: Criterion-related validity of the Diagnostic Criteria for Psychosomatic Research for alexithymia in patients with functional gastrointestinal disorders. Psychother Psychosom 2001;70:184–188.
66 Lumley MA, Stettner L, Wehmer F: How are alexithymia and physical illness linked? A review and critique of pathways. J Psychosom Res 1996;41:505–518.
67 Kellner R: Psychosomatic Syndromes and Somatic Symptoms. Washington, American Psychiatric Press, 1991.
68 Kroenke K, Spitzer RL, DeFruy FV, Hahn SR, Linzer M, Williams JBW, Brody D, Davis M: Multisomatoform disorder. An alternative to undifferentiated somatoform disorder for the somatizing patient in primary care. Arch Gen Psychiatry 1997;54:352–358.
69 Bridges KW, Goldberg DP: Somatic presentation of DSM-III psychiatric disorders in primary care. J Psychosom Res 1985;29:563–569.
70 Karlsson H, Joukamaa M, Lahti I, Lehtinen V, Kokki-Saarinen T: Frequent attender profiles: different clinical subgroups among frequent attender patients in primary care. J Psychosom Res 1997;42:157–166.
71 Barsky AJ, Klerman GL: Overview: hypochondriasis, bodily complaints and somatic styles. Am J Psychiatry 1983;140:273–283.
72 Bartolucci G, Savron G, Fava GA, Grandi S, Trombini G, Orlandi C: Psychological reactions to thermography and mammography. Stress Med 1989;5:195–199.
73 Grandi S: The sequential parallel comparison model: a revolution in the design of clinical trials. Psychother Psychosom 2003;72:113–114.
74 Fava M, Evins AE, Dorer DJ, Schoenfeld DA: The problem of the placebo response in clinical trials for psychiatric disorders: culprits, possible remedies, and a novel study design approach. Psychother Psychosom 2003;72:115–127.
75 Pitz M, Cheang M, Bernstein CN: Defining the predictors of the placebo response in irritable bowel syndrome. Clin Gastroenterol Hepat 2005;3:237–247.
76 Mearin F, Balboa A, Zarate N, Cucala M, Malagelada JR: Placebo in functional dyspepsia: symptomatic, gastrointestinal motor, and gastric sensorial responses. Am J Gastroenterol 1999;94:116–125.

77 Vandvik PO, Wilhelmsen I, Ihlebaek C, Farup PG: Comorbidity of irritable bowel syndrome in general practice: a striking feature with clinical implications. Aliment Pharmacol Ther 2004;20: 1195–1203.
78 Porcelli P, De Carne M, Fava GA: Assessing somatization in functional gastrointestinal disorders: integration of different criteria. Psychother Psychosom 2000;69:198–204.

Dr. Piero Porcelli
Unità di Psicosomatica, IRCCS Ospedale De Bellis
Via della Resistenza
IT–70013 Castellana Grotte (Italy)
Tel. +39 080 499 4685, Fax +39 080 499 4340, E-Mail porcellip@media.it

Porcelli P, Sonino N (eds): Psychological Factors Affecting Medical Conditions. A New Classification for DSM-V. Adv Psychosom Med. Basel, Karger, 2007, vol 28, pp 57–71

Psychological Factors Affecting Oncology Conditions

Luigi Grassi[a,b], *Bruno Biancosino*[b], *Luciana Marmai*[b], *Elena Rossi*[a,b], *Silvana Sabato*[a,b]

[a]Section of Psychiatry, Department of Medical Sciences of Communication and Behavior, University of Ferrara, [b]Clinical Psychiatry Unit, Department of Mental Health, Health Organization of Ferrara and S. Anna University Hospital, Ferrara, Italy

Abstract

The area of psychological factors affecting cancer has been the object of research starting from the early 1950s and consolidating from the 1970s with the development of psycho-oncology. A series of problems in the DSM and ICD nosological systems, such as the difficult application of the criteria for psychiatric diagnoses (i.e. major depression, adjustment disorders) and the scarce space dedicated to the rubric of psychosocial implications of medical illness (i.e. Psychological Factors Affecting a Medical Condition under 'Other Conditions That May Be a Focus of Clinical Attention' in the DSM-IV) represent a major challenge in psycho-oncology. The application of the Diagnostic Criteria for Psychosomatic Research (DCPR) has been shown to be useful in a more precise identification of several psychological domains in patients with cancer. The DCPR dimensions of health anxiety, demoralization and alexithymia have been shown to be quite frequent in cancer patient (37.7, 28.8 and 26%, respectively). The overlap between a formal DSM-IV diagnosis and the DCPR is low, with 58% of patients being categorized as non-cases on the DSM-IV having at least one DCPR syndrome. The specific quality of the DCPR in characterizing psychosocial aspects secondary to cancer is also confirmed by the fact that some dimensions of coping (e.g. Mini-Mental Adjustment to Cancer subscale hopelessness) correlate with the DCPR dimension of demoralization, while a quantitative approach on symptom assessment (e.g. stress symptoms on the Brief Symptom Inventory) is not useful in discriminating the patients with and without DCPR syndromes. More research is needed in order to understand the relationship between DCPR constructs (e.g. alexithymia) and psychosocial factors which have been shown to be significant in oncology (e.g. emotional repression and avoidance). The role of specific DCPR constructs in influencing the course of illness is also an area that should be investigated.

Cancer is one of the most common diseases worldwide and it is the second leading cause of death [1]. According to the World Health Organization, 15 million people have been newly diagnosed as having cancer and almost 8 million people died of cancer in 2005, and more than 20 million people in the world are living with cancer. The incidence of cancer has increased from 1950 to 2005 as a result of a rapidly ageing population in many countries, and an increased exposure to cancer risk factors such as tobacco use, unhealthy diet, physical inactivity, some infections, and carcinogens. These figures are extremely clear in explaining the reasons why the evaluation and understanding of the psychosocial variables related to cancer and its treatments has been the focus of psychiatric and psychosomatic literature since the 1950s.

The first approach was based on what the psychosomatic movement had proposed as a psychoanalytic formulation of medical illness. In this context, it was suggested that early family dynamics, traumatic events, unconscious sexual conflicts and personality traits were etiologically linked with the onset of cancer [2, 3]. As reported by Holland [4], this approach later branched into two areas relevant to cancer, one related to the series of studies in the area of psychobiology of stress (e.g. psychoneuroendocrinology, psychoneuroimmunology), the second related to the development of consultation-liaison psychiatry. This second area gradually prevailed in the literature starting from the 1970s, with clinicians more interested in understanding how to help cancer patients and their families, rather than in speculating on psychological causes of cancer. In fact, unlike psychodynamic formulation, the psychological response of patients with cancer, the effects of treatments on social roles and return to work, the effects of psychiatric disorders or maladaptive coping styles on the patients' quality of life, interpersonal relationships, adherence to treatment and possibly prognosis were close to the experience of oncologists and health care professionals involved in cancer care.

On these bases, the development and the diffusion of psycho-oncology (it does not matter if considered by some as a subspecialty of oncology, by others as a subspecialty of consultation-liaison psychiatry or psychosomatic medicine) in the last 20 years has made clear the need to consider the multiple psychosocial implications of cancer as an integral part of cancer care, with the mission that all cancer patients and their families throughout the world receive optimal psychosocial care at all stages of disease and survivorship [5].

General Psychosocial Implications of Cancer

Starting form a biopsychosocial approach, the consequences of cancer diagnosis and treatment (surgery, chemotherapy, radiotherapy, hormone therapy) are extremely significant.

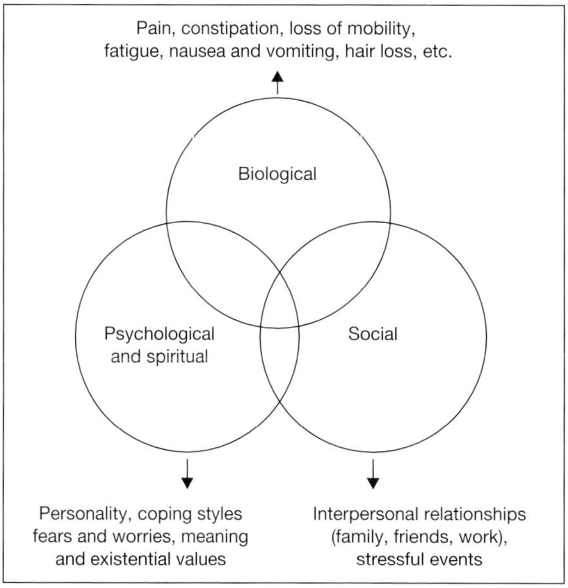

Fig. 1. The interplay of factors in the biopsychosocial approach to cancer.

At the physical level, cancer can cause significant changes in the body and consequently the image the individual has of his own body. The type of cancer ('visible' cancers, like breast cancer, or 'less visible' cancer, like leukemia), its stage, its biological characteristics and the effects of treatment (e.g. physical mutilations, stomas, pain, nausea and vomiting, hair loss, fatigue) are important in determining the different emotional responses of the patients. Functional activity, feeling of dependency from others, sexuality, are only examples of the somatic and biological concomitants of cancer and cancer treatments. From the psychological point of view, the loss of certainties, instability of one's own emotional state (e.g. fears, anxiety, worries, sadness), change of perspective in the future and threat of possible death and dying are only some of the numerous experiences cancer patients have to deal with during the trajectory of illness. At a spiritual level, the meaning that human beings give to their life (e.g. personal values, the meaning of time and being, transcendence) are further areas to be considered. The interpersonal level is a also touched by cancer and cancer treatment, since the sense of belonging (to be with, to communicate as to put in common with someone) in the family, in the microcosm of close relationships and in the macrocosm of society (e.g. work, social activity, policy) is also threatened by cancer. Possible feelings of loneliness, abandonment, anomia, marginalization or even stigmatization are problems that cancer patients should deal with during their trajectory of illness (fig. 1).

These factors fluctuate during the different phases of the disease (diagnosis, active treatment, discharge from the hospital, follow-up, surviving cancer, palliative care) and its course (remission, recurrence, progression and end of life) with psychosocial implications changing over time.

Clinical Implications of the Psychosocial Dimensions in Cancer Patients

The importance of these aspects has been taken into consideration by consultation-liaison psychiatry and psycho-oncology studies. It should be noted that the majority of studies tried to examine the impact of the above-described psychosocial dimensions in favoring the onset of psychiatric disorders. A bulk of data showed that of 40–50% of cancer patients, in any phase of illness, can be diagnosed as having a psychiatric diagnosis according to the DSM-IV or ICD-10 criteria, such as adjustment disorders, major depression, and posttraumatic stress disorders [5]. However, the application of the usual criteria used in psychiatry showed to be problematic, both for their low specificity and sensitivity and the need to modify and adapt the diagnostic criteria of several psychiatric diagnoses. Furthermore, the largest area of emotional reactions, including distress, anger, denial and other psychosocial dimensions and/or conditions is extremely important in oncology.

In fact, a series of studies have shown that psychosocial factors, other than psychiatric diagnoses, have a remarkable role in negatively influencing the patients' quality of life, their interpersonal relationships, behavioral dimensions (e.g. adherence to treatment, maladaptive coping and maintenance of at-risk behavior) and possibly prognosis and survival. Grassi et al. [6] and Grassi and Rosti [7] have shown that, among cancer patients, a series of attitudes and perceptions of health status, subsumed under the concept of abnormal illness behavior (e.g. affective inhibition, disease conviction in spite of medical reassurance, frictions in interpersonal relationships, inability to perceive the role of psychological factors in symptom perceptions) are related to depressive states, not necessarily meeting the criteria of a DSM or ICD psychiatric disorder. Furthermore, maladaptive coping styles, such as hopelessness-helplessness and anxious preoccupation, have been related to other psychosocial dimensions, including poor social support and personality variables, such as external locus of control, irrespective of a formal psychiatric diagnosis [8]. The dimension of demoralization, as a clinical syndrome separated from major depression has been shown to be extremely common and important in cancer settings, even though it cannot be correctly detected by psychiatric nosographic systems [9].

The role of psychological factors in molding the course of cancer has also been studied. In a prospective study of 578 breast cancer patients, it has been shown that hopelessness response (rather than a formal diagnosis of major depression) is implicated in increasing the risk of relapse or death at both 5 years after diagnosis and 10 years later [10, 11]. A different study carried out in patients with locoregional breast cancer showed that cancer survival is affected by a complex combination of psychosocial factors, among which minimizing was found to predict a favorable prognosis and anger repression (nonexpression) and escape behavior an unfavorable prognosis [12]. Similar data on the role of minimization in increasing survival of metastatic breast cancer patients were reported by Butow et al. [13]. Low levels of psychological distress, low fatigue and lack of anxiety independently predicted longer recurrence-free and overall survival, controlling for biological factors, among 1,588 breast cancer patients at an average time of 12 years after diagnosis [14]. The role of psychological factors in molding the prognosis has also been shown in a study of lung cancer patients in which interviewer-rated emotional distress was significantly associated with shorter survival, independent of the influence of the biomedical prognostic factors [15], and in a study of patients with metastatic melanoma [16] in which minimization and anger were independently predictive of survival over time.

Current Evaluation of Psychological Factors Affecting a Medical Condition

According to these data, the assessment of the different psychosocial dimensions in medically ill patients, and specifically in cancer patients should be a routine approach in clinical care. A number of psychometric instruments have been proposed and are available with regard to this. However, the risk of reducing the complex subjective and experiential dimensions in multiple-choice instruments has been raised by Fava et al. [17], who consider more structured and clinical approach as the necessary way to overcome the problem of reductionism in medicine. On the other hand, in a more articulated clinical tool such as the DSM-IV [18], a short rubric is dedicated to this vast area ('Psychological Factors Affecting a Medical Condition') under the chapter 'Other Conditions That May Be a Focus of Clinical Attention'. Likewise, the ICD-10 [19] summarizes this area in chapter 21 under the rubric 'Factors Influencing Health Status and Contact with Health System' (code Z00-Z99).

According to the DSM-IV (table 1), psychological or behavioral factors may adversely affect cancer, as well as almost every general medical condition, in different ways. They may influence the course of cancer, interfere with treatment

Table 1. Diagnostic criteria for psychological factor affecting cancer (adapted from DSM-IV-TR) [18]

A. A general medical condition (coded on axis III) is present

B. Psychological factors adversely affect the general medical condition in one of the following ways:
   (1) The factors have influenced the course of the general medical condition as shown by a close temporal association between the psychological factors and the development or exacerbation of, or delayed recovery from, the general medical condition
   (2) The factors interfere with the treatment of the general medical condition
   (3) The factors constitute additional health risks for the individual
   (4) Stress-related physiological responses precipitate or exacerbate symptoms of the general medical condition

It is necessary to indicate the nature of the psychological factors (if more than one factor is present, indicate the most prominent):

Mental disorder affecting cancer (e.g. an axis I disorder such as major depressive disorder delaying recovery from surgery after cancer or influencing psychoneuroimmunological pathways)

Psychological symptoms affecting cancer (e.g. depressive symptoms delaying recovery from surgery or reducing adherence to treatment, such as hormone therapy, chemotherapy, radiotherapy)

Personality traits or coping style affecting cancer (e.g. pathological denial of the need for surgery in a patient with cancer)

Maladaptive health behaviors affecting cancer (e.g. smoking; poor or unbalanced diet; lack of exercise; exposure to risk factors for cancer)

Stress-related physiological response affecting cancer (e.g. stress-related exacerbations of pain, nausea, vomiting)

Other or unspecified psychological factors affecting cancer (e.g. interpersonal, cultural, or religious factors)

of cancer, constitute an additional health risk for the individual, precipitate or exacerbate symptoms by eliciting stress-related physiological responses (e.g. pain, nausea and vomiting).

The psychological or behavioral factors that influence cancer include axis I disorders, axis II disorders, psychological symptoms or personality traits that do not meet the full criteria for a specific mental disorder, maladaptive health behaviors, or physiological responses to environmental or social stressors.

From the DSM-IV criteria, it derives that there must be reasonable evidence to suggest an association between the psychological factors and cancer. In other words, psychological factors should have a clinically significant effect on the course or outcome of the general medical condition or place the individual at a significantly higher risk for an adverse outcome, although it is not always possible to demonstrate direct causality or the mechanisms underlying the relationship. From the clinical point of view, psychological and behavioral factors can be represented by an axis I disorder (e.g. major depression), personality traits or coping styles (e.g. high hostility levels in the relationship with the staff, coping styles based on giving-up and resignation), maladaptive health behaviors (e.g. sedentary lifestyle, continued smoking, excessive alcohol use), stress-related physiological responses (e.g. tension increasing the experience of pain, anxiety favoring chemotherapy-related nausea).

Some problems arise in this classification, however. First, an overlapping between psychiatric diagnoses and psychosocial dimensions is evident (axis I, personality traits and maladaptive coping). Furthermore, no specific explanation is given about how to assess the dimensions mentioned, indicating that more detailed examination of the different psychosocial dimensions involved in medically ill patient is needed.

Development of the Diagnostic Criteria for Psychosomatic Research and Its Application in Cancer Settings

The development of the Diagnostic Criteria for Psychosomatic Research (DCPR) has provided new insight in this area. The DCPR are a series of syndromes specifically developed by an international group of investigators [20, 21] to translate psychosocial variables that were derived from psychosomatic research into operational tools whereby medially ill patients can be identified. The DCPR consist of 12 clinical categories – or clusters – which, through a semistructured interview, explore a variety of possible psychological conditions and emotional responses to medical illness. These are represented by eight clusters dealing with the concept of abnormal illness behavior (health anxiety, irritable mood, demoralization, illness denial, alexithymia, type a behavior, thanatophobia, disease phobia) and four dealing with somatoform disorders (functional somatic symptoms secondary to a psychiatric disorder, persistent somatization, conversion syndrome, anniversary reaction).

Interesting and clinically useful results emerged in the application of the DCPR in oncology. In a study of 146 patients with a diagnosis of cancer within 18 months and a good performance status, who were evaluated by using both the DSM-IV and the DCPR, Grassi et al. [22] have indicated that 44.5% subjects (n = 65) met the criteria for a DSM-IV diagnosis (DSM cases), mainly adjustment disorders (28%) and mood disorders (10.3%), while 71.2% presented symptoms meeting the criteria for at least one DCPR syndrome. The most frequent DCPR dimensions were health anxiety (37.7%), demoralization (28.8%) and alexithymia (26%). A lower percentage of patients reported irritable mood (11.6%), type A behavior (9.5%), thanatophobia (8.2%) and illness denial (8.2%). DSM-IV and DCPR diagnoses were neither related to the stage of illness nor the type of treatment received (i.e. chemotherapy and radiotherapy).

The authors showed an overlap between DSM-IV and DCPR diagnoses for only 57 patients (39% of the total sample and 50.9% of those with DCPR or

DSM diagnoses). Among those who had no formal DSM-IV psychiatric diagnosis (n = 81, 55.5%), 47 received a DCPR diagnosis (58% false negatives; 39.2% of the total sample). Only 8 patients with a DSM-IV diagnosis (adjustment disorder, n = 7; personality disorder, n = 1) were not identified by the DCPR (5.5% of the total sample, 12.3% of those with a DSM-IV diagnosis). A further interesting result was that the intensity of distress symptoms was not useful in detecting patients with DCPR psychosocial syndromes. In fact, by using the Brief Symptom Inventory, which provides scores of emotional stress in several dimensions (e.g. anxiety, depression, hostility, interpersonal sensitivity, general stress), the scores were higher among DSM-IV cases but not among patients with a DCPR syndrome.

In a different study of 105 breast cancer patients who underwent the DCPR semistructured interview, the same authors [23] showed that 38.1% subjects presented symptoms meeting the criteria for at least one DCPR syndrome and a further 28.6% had more than one DCPR syndrome. Health anxiety (38.1%), demoralization (28.6%), alexithymia (20%) and irritable mood (14.3%) were the most commonly reported DCPR constellations, while the remaining DCPR dimensions were positive in a lower percentage of subjects (irritable mood, 14.3%; type A behavior, 10.5%; illness denial, 9.5%; thanatophobia, 5.7%). In general, the patients with DCPR syndromes reported higher levels of sadness, more physical symptoms, poorer well-being, poorer leisure activity and lower support from interpersonal ties, as subjectively measured by using a 0–10 Visual Analogue Scale, than women without any DCPR syndrome. The two groups were also different in terms of worries and preoccupation related to cancer (e.g. the illness itself, the effects of treatment, feeling different from others, the impact on sexual life, the future), as evaluated using the Cancer Worry Inventory. Patients who were positive on the DCPR showed higher scores on the Cancer Worry Inventory than patients without any DCPR syndrome. Interesting data were reported when examining the relationship between the single DCPR dimensions and coping styles, as measured by the Mini-Mental Adjustment to Cancer Scale (Mini-MAC), a questionnaire specifically devised to explore coping style in cancer patients (e.g. fighting spirit, fatalism, anxious preoccupation, hopelessness, avoidance). The patients positive on the health anxiety dimension reported higher scores on the Mini-MAC anxious preoccupation subscale, which indicates the presence of feelings of anxiety and tension concerning the illness (e.g. 'I worry about the cancer returning or getting worse'; 'I am frightened'). Those meeting the criteria demoralization had higher scores on the Mini-MAC hopelessness subscale, which indicates the presence of the patient's tendency to adopt a pessimistic and hopeless-helpless attitude towards his/her illness (e.g. 'I feel that life is hopeless'; 'I feel like giving up'; 'I feel there is nothing I can do to help myself'). Finally, patients meeting the DCPR cluster of alexithymia had higher scores on the Mini-MAC avoidance subscale, which indicates the presence of a coping style characterized by a tendency to avoid confrontation with illness (e.g. 'I make a positive effort not to think about my illness'; 'I distract myself when thoughts about my illness come into my head'; 'I deliberately push all thoughts of cancer out of my mind').

Somatization in Cancer: A Further Application of the DCPR

Alongside with the data presented, the DCPR might give some important information on the dimensions of somatization which have never been examined until now by application of this system in oncology. In general, this is a complex area in patients affected by a demonstrated medical illness and, as far as oncology is concerned, somatization in cancer has often been overlooked or completely ignored, mainly due to the presumption that if somatic symptoms occur in a patient with cancer, these are due to the disease itself and/or its progression. However, complaints of tiredness, fatigue, poor concentration and irritability, likely related to psychological factors, are frequently reported by cancer patients. Data regarding abnormal illness behavior and somatization have been reported by a few studies carried out in oncology. Hypochondriasis, a high tendency to evaluate in somatic terms bodily functions and somatization were shown to be unchanged in patients who recovered from cancer and who were evaluated at the time of the diagnosis and 6 years later in a prospective study carried out by our group [24]. Results in line with these findings were also reported in a study of 98 consecutive patients referred for psychiatric consultation by Chaturvedi et al. [25]. The authors showed that 28% had prominent somatic presentation with multiple somatic symptoms confirming an association between somatization, depressed mood, and cancer. Common somatic complaints in this study were pain (19%), fatigue (17%), sensory symptoms (30%) and mixed symptoms (27%). More recently, Carlson et al. [26] reported a high prevalence of psychological distress in cancer patients (37%) and among patients with psychological distress, somatization, followed by depression and anxiety, were the most frequent reported symptoms.

The importance of this clinical and research area has been recently underlined by Chaturvedi et al. [27], who indicated that somatic symptoms magnify disability resulting from cancer, interfere with treatment adherence and decisions, cause delay in recovery, result in poor outcome and recurrence, and reduce overall well-being and quality of life. Secondly, somatic symptoms in cancer may complicate the diagnosis of major depression due to the overlap of symptoms occurring as a result of the underlying disease, depression or somatoform disorder. Furthermore, somatic symptoms in cancer are unique in being interrelated with each other, with one somatic symptom causing other somatic symptoms (for example, pain causing fatigue). It is a difficult task to identify the exact etiology of somatic symptoms in cancer patients, which may be due to different factors: physical, psychological or both. In a controlled study [28], it was observed that somatization in disease-free cancer patients was related to anxiety and depression. Cancer patients with somatization also had excessive somatic concern and preoccupation, but whether this is the cause or effect of suffering from persistent somatic symptoms is difficult to conclude. It could be the effect of persistent somatization since most subjects had no previous evidence of somatization. Depressive symptoms and depressive disorders were encountered commonly in these patients, and this association between depression and somatization is similar to that documented in psychiatric populations. Assessment of somatic symptoms and differentiation of their etiology need careful evaluation of the association with stress and psychological factors. When somatic symptoms arise or aggravate after stress, psychological or emotional factors, they are likely to be psychological somatic symptoms. Those related to progression of disease or treatments are clearly physical. Some somatic symptoms may have both physical and psychological factors implicated. Lastly, there may be somatic symptoms which may not be clearly physical or psychological in origin and may be idiopathic. The application of the DCPR alongside with a careful investigation of the history of the patient, as recommended in the assessment of somatization in clinical practice [29], can be of extreme help in better understanding this clinical area in patients affected by cancer, mainly in those with the early stage of cancer, after completion of treatment and patients with long survival.

Discussion

The development of the DCPR has been followed by a series of clinical studies showing that this system can facilitate the identification of psychological syndromes (e.g. demoralization, type A behavior, irritable mood and alexithymia), which are not recognized by the DSM-IV, in patients with different types of medical illness such as gastrointestinal disorders [30], heart disease [31, 32], endocrine diseases [33], and dermatological disorders [34]. With respect to this and according to the experience we have collected, the DCPR represent a promising approach and a useful tool also in the oncology setting. Several implications can be discussed with regard to how the DCPR can allow clinicians to have significant information on the psychosocial concomitants secondary to cancer.

A first general consideration is that through the DCPR it is possible to identify psychosocial dimensions formally undiagnosed by the DSM-IV alone.

Furthermore the specification of the phenomenology of these dimensions can be reached by using the DCPR interview which is able to give precise information of the patients' psychological problems. This is not easy or possible at all by using the general rubric of 'Psychological Factors Affecting a Medical Condition' of the DSM-IV. It is that the DSM-V may take advantage of the literature emerged in this area, including the research related to the use of the DCPR, and may improve the conceptualization of this chapter with the benefit of the clinical approach to medical illnesses.

A second and more specific consideration regards the characterization of these dimensions in cancer patients, given the need for a precise assessment of psychological factors that may negatively influence coping with illness and mental health [35]. From what we presented, it has been shown that health anxiety, demoralization, and alexithymia are the most frequent DCPR syndromes. These results support the psycho-oncology literature that has focused attention on demoralization, giving up and hopelessness and avoidance/emotional repression as significant dimensions to be considered in cancer patients. Regarding demoralization, its phenomenological expression and the difference between major depression and demoralization have been pointed out by some authors [36]. Through the use of the DCPR among medically ill patients, it has been confirmed that demoralization is a construct that is not necessarily related to major depression and that it should be examined carefully, avoiding the common tendency to dismiss it as an understandable (and thus not requiring treatment) condition in patients with medical illnesses [37]. How the DCPR construct of demoralization fits with other constructs of demoralization should be examined, however. Kissane [38] and Clarke and Kissane [39] have extensively studied demoralization and indicated the importance of the demoralization syndrome as a distinct psychiatric condition in which loss of meaning and hope can determine a sense of worthlessness on one's own life and in the future. The authors have proposed some criteria for the diagnosis of demoralization [9] and have also developed a scale to measure it in clinical settings [40]. The DCPR and the criteria for the demoralization syndrome are presented in table 2.

The relationship of demoralization and hopelessness should also be investigated in cancer patients [41]. In fact, hopelessness, rather than major depression according the DSM-IV, was found to be a significant factor implicated in suicidal ideation and wish to die among cancer patients [42] and one of the key elements in the relationship between individual psychosocial response and cancer progression [10, 11, 43]. From the psychobiological point of view, Argaman et al. [44] have hypothesized that hopelessness may negatively influence the outcome of cancer via interleukin-1β (IL-1β). A series of data could be in line with this hypothesis, specifically the fact that IL-1β is elevated in the brain following exposure to inescapable shock, that hopelessness is minimized by antagonizing

Table 2. The diagnosis of demoralization according to the DCPR [20] and the demoralization syndrome [9]

DCPR	Demoralization syndrome
1. Feelings of having failed to meet one's own expectations or those of other people (concerning work, family, social and/or economic status) 2. Inability to cope with some pressing problems 3. Feelings of helplessness, hopelessness, and/or giving up 4. This state has been prolonged and generalized (exceeding at least 1 month) 5. This state closely antedated the manifestation of a physical disorder or exacerbates it	1. Affective symptoms of existential distress including hopelessness or loss of meaning and purpose in life 2. Cognitive attitudes of pessimism, helplessness, sense of being trapped, personal failure, or lacking a worthwhile future 3. Conative absence of drive or motivation to cope differently 4. Associated features of social alienation or isolation and lack of support 5. Allowing for fluctuation in emotional intensity, these phenomena persist across more than 2 weeks 6. A major depressive episode or other psychiatric is not present as the primary condition

cerebral IL-1β, that elevated cerebral IL-1β increases cancer metastasis in animals.

Regarding the DCPR construct of alexithymia and its relationship with other psychological factors or coping mechanisms, such as avoidance, more data are needed. From one perspective, the component of difficulty identifying feelings of the alexithymia construct was significantly higher in cancer patients experiencing pain [45]. From another perspective, it has been shown that alexithymia and repressive coping style are associated with impairments in the recognition of both pleasant and unpleasant emotions, such as anger or happiness [46]. At the same time, suppression of emotions has been related to higher levels of psychological distress in cancer patients [47, 48]. The meaning of alexithymia in cancer patients (e.g. primary or secondary alexithymia) and its effect have not been clarified. Also, the difference between cancer patients and the general population is not known, considering that alexithymic traits have been reported in a high percentage of healthy people in a study of a community sample [49].

A third and last consideration of the DCPR application in oncology has to do with the role of psychometric instruments in assessing psychosocial dimensions of cancer. In relation to the screening instruments for distress, such as the

corticotrophin-releasing factor. This stimulation leads to hyperactivity of the hypothalamic-pituitary-adrenal axis and high plasma cortisol levels. Depression is also associated with stimulation of the sympathetic nervous system, which is associated with elevated levels of circulating plasma norepinephrine levels [64]. Such stimulation is associated with resultant dysfunction of the autonomic nervous system. Depressed subjects generally manifest increases in resting heart rates compared with nondepressed controls and decreased heart rate variability in some cohorts with depression, as well baroreflex dysfunction and increased QT variability as an index of ventricular repolarization dishomogeneity. Depression or related emotional states are also associated with complex platelet abnormalities (in activation, secretion and aggregation) such as increased concentrations of functional glycoprotein IIb/IIIa receptors [65] and hyperactivity of the 5-hydroxytryptamine $transporter_{2A}$ receptor signal transduction system [66]. Furthermore, there is new research into the evolving understanding of how depression can promote inflammation and the link between inflammation and atherosclerosis (potentially bidirectional). Depression is also linked to a range of immune abnormalities, including increased production of cytokines and acute-phase proteins such as C-reactive protein [67].

Demoralization

Recently, prospective epidemiological studies have also reported a relationship between symptoms of hopelessness and the development of CHD through carotid atherosclerosis [68, 69]. A related phenomenon is 'vital exhaustion'. Appels and Mulder [70] found that this state, characterized by unusual fatigue, increased irritability and demoralized feelings, is associated with an increased risk of MI. Schmale and Engel [71] have provided a detailed account for demoralization, which they defined as the 'giving up-given up complex'. Such a subsyndromal state cannot be identified with psychiatric categories [72]. The DCPR [5] identify a syndrome characterized by the patient's consciousness of having failed to meet his or her own expectations or those of others or being unable to cope with some pressing problems. The patient experiences feelings of helplessness, or hopelessness or giving up. In the cited study by Rafanelli et al. [11], DCPR were used to detect demoralization: 20% of patients were identified as suffering from demoralization 1 year before the first episode of MI or angina. In 12% of patients, there was an overlap between major depression and demoralization. Demoralization could not be considered a cardiac risk factor per se, but the addition of this subsyndromal state to major depression could individuate a subgroup of patients at a greater risk of a cardiac morbidity [11]. In the cited study by Ottolini et al. [24] at least one DCPR diagnosis was found in all patients; 51% of patients reported demoralization; 14.8%

was the overlap rate of DCPR demoralization with DSM-IV mood disorders. There is a phenomenological ground whereby demoralization can be differentiated from major depression [73, 74]. In fact, in the samples of the cited studies [11, 24], the subjects who had a mood disorder did not necessarily present demoralization and vice versa. The diagnostic criteria for demoralization attempt to capture the state of feeling that Schmale and Engel [71] outlined as a facilitating factor for the onset of disease to which the individual was predisposed. This factor thus likely decreases individual vulnerability to disease. The results of the study by Rafanelli et al. [11] and Ottolini et al. [24] lend support to the importance of assessing both clinical and subclinical symptoms. Using DCPR [14], the authors outlined a more specific profile which seems to be characteristic of MI patients.

Irritable Mood

The experience of irritability is part of the normal human repertoire. Everyday stresses, such as noise, traffic, a long wait, a rude answer, may elicit irritable mood [75]. A substantial problem of research on irritability lies in the various ways it is defined [76]. Slater and Roth [77] defined irritability as a mode of response to psychological stimuli of a particular kind, such as those in which the individual is threatened in some way, or is frustrated in a purposive course of action. A considerable body of evidence has suggested a pathogenetic role for anger, hostility and irritable mood in physical illness, both of organic and functional nature [77]. The DCPR definition of irritable mood [5], a feeling state which requires an increased effort of control over temper by the individual or results in irascible verbal or behavioral outbursts, is largely based on the work of Snaith and Taylor [78]. It may be experienced as brief episodes, in particular circumstances, or it may be prolonged and generalized. Irritability can covary but differs from depressed mood. It may be part of the type A personality associated with hostile cynicism. In the cited study by Ottolini et al. [24], irritable mood was the most frequent DCPR diagnosis (56% of the patients) retrospectively investigated in a sample of 92 patients at first episode of MI. This syndrome was frequently associated with anxiety disorders.

Health Anxiety

A major problem with the DSM-IV classification of hypochondriacal fears and attitudes is that they only define the most severe end of the spectrum (hypochondriasis, characterized by resistance to medical reassurance and multiple fears). There is evidence [79, 80] that other worries are worthy of clinical attention, such as health anxiety, indicating preoccupations about health in the absence of a pathology or excessive concern in case pathology is present. The main aspect of health anxiety seems to be the presence of dysfunctional beliefs about health and illnesses which could derive from past experiences of illness in oneself or others [81, 82]. These worries are part of a vicious circle characterized by selective perception and misinterpretation of bodily symptoms which all together may increase health anxiety. DCPR [5] define health anxiety as generic worry about illness, concern about pain and bodily preoccupations (tendency to amplify somatic sensations). Worries and fears are characterized as readily responding to appropriate medical reassurance, even though new worries may ensue after some time. Health anxiety was one of the most frequent diagnostic finding and accounted for 41% of the total sample in the study by Ottolini et al. [24]. Health anxiety was frequently associated with mood disorders.

Type A Behavior

The belief that a pattern of aggressive or irascible behavior is associated with CHD holds a peculiar and persistent fascination for both the lay public and physicians and psychologists [83]. While the history of the idea can be traced back for at least several centuries, the scientific study of the possible behavioral basis of CHD was laid by the pioneering work of Friedman and Rosenman, who, over 30 years ago, described what they termed the type A or coronary prone behavior pattern [84, 85]. This pattern was characterized by hard driving and competitive behavior, ambition, drive for success, a potential for hostility, a subjective sense of time urgency, devotion to work, restlessness, pronounced impatience, and vigorous speech stylistic and abruptness of gesture [22, 83]. Type A behavior is exhibited by persons who are constantly engaged in a struggle to achieve, to outdo others, and to meet deadlines. It is not synonymous with life stress, nor does it represent a response to life stress. Rather, it constitutes a habitual behavioral state whose precursors have been observed in children [22]. It seems that type A behavior represents specific manifest features of an interaction between a set of psychological characteristics and specific stimulus situations that provoke them and promote their full expression (the social environment that offers opportunities and rewards for competitive striving and a related value system, the easy access to a diet rich in saturated fats and calories, tobacco and transportation) [22]. Type A behavior was measured using a mildly challenging structured interview and it was determined both from the content of the subject's answers to the interview questions and also from the style in which they responded. A large number of studies have been conducted in the past 3 decades on the pathogenic role of type A behavior [86] in CHD [87]. Various methods of assessment have been used and the results have been rather controversial. A substantial problem of psychosomatic research in this field has been the fact of using dimensional instruments and postulating the presence of type A behavior pattern in every cardiac patient [14]. The most relevant clinical features of DCPR type A behavior pattern [5], such as excessive degree of involvement in work and pervasive sense of time urgency, elicit stress-related physiologic responses that precipitate or exacerbate symptoms of the medical condition. On the basis of early positive findings in the Framingham study [88] and the Western Collaborative Group's 8-year follow-up [89], among other evidence, the National Institutes of Health declared type A an independent risk factor for CHD. However, with the publication of negative findings [90–92] it was proposed that more specific components of type A, namely hostility and time urgency, might be key components [87], although there are conflicting studies due to inadequacies of measurement [83]. In the study by Ottolini et al. [24], 40% of the patients presented type A behavior detected by DCPR. Type A behavior was frequently associated with anxiety disorders. The results indicate that not all cardiac patients present with type A behavior. In those who do, the onset of irritable mood may interact with type A personality characteristics to increase psychosomatic vulnerability. In those who do not present type A features, the clinical development of symptoms may be different. Unlike other psychosocial factors, type A is distinguished by being the subject of numerous intervention trials [93].

Cardiac Rehabilitation

Cardiac rehabilitation (CR) programs have been found to play an important part in improving recovery, quality of life and in decreasing mortality [94–98]. They typically include components of physical training, modification of lifestyle, pharmacological treatment and psychological counseling.

DSM Syndromes

The aim of a study by Rafanelli et al. [14] was to document the prevalence of psychological distress in a consecutive sample of patients undergoing a CR program. A consecutive series of 61 patients with recent (within 1 month), first MI who were referred to a CR program was included in the study. Assessment included a modified version of the Structured Clinical Interview for eliciting psychiatric diagnoses [99] according to DSM-IV criteria [100]; also the diagnosis of minor depression was included. The CR program of the hospital extends over 4 weeks and includes the following components: individualized physical training program and tailored intervention on cardiovascular risk factors (arterial hypertension, hypercholesterolemia, diabetes mellitus and smoking habits). Twelve of 61 patients (20%) received a psychiatric diagnosis. Minor depression was present in 9.8% of the cases, social phobia in 4.9%, agoraphobia without panic attacks in 3.3%, major depression in 1.6% and blood-injury phobia in

1.6%. The DSM-IV diagnosis of minor depression was used in this study and accounted for most of the psychiatric diagnoses. Had this been excluded, as is common in clinical practice, the results with DSM would have been even more disappointing. In contrast to unselected samples of patients with recent MI, depression was not a common psychiatric disorder. There was only 1 case of major depressive disorder and demoralization and another 8 of minor depression or demoralization. Depressive symptoms have been linked to CR and outcome [101]. It is thus conceivable that the presence of depression and/or demoralization could prevent patients from participating in the program. In our sample, it was found that anxiety disorders may play a role in the CR programs.

Another study by Rafanelli et al. [102] assessed, by the same reliable methods of the previous study [14], clinical distress in a consecutive sample of patients who underwent CABG. One month after CABG, at the first psychological assessment during the CR program, 17 (36.1%) of 47 patients received a psychiatric diagnosis. The prevalence of mood disorders was 23.4%: 6 patients (12.8%) reported minor depression; 5 (10.6%) major depression; 3 patients (6.4%) reported agoraphobia; 2 (4.3%) social phobia; 2 (4.3%) undifferentiated somatoform disorder; 1 (2.1%) an obsessive compulsive disorder.

DCPR Syndromes

In the cited study by Rafanelli et al. [14], the semistructured interview, based on a preliminary instrument [103] for subclinical psychological syndromes, the DCPR [5] were also used. Twenty-three of the 61 patients (38%) had a DCPR cluster, with a total of 31 DCPR diagnoses. There was overlap between the two classification (DSM and DCPR) systems. Five of the 12 patients with DSM-IV diagnoses had an associated DCPR cluster. In 18 cases, therefore, there was a DCPR cluster without any associated psychiatric diagnosis (30%). Altogether, about half of the patients received either a DSM or DCPR diagnosis. The most striking finding was the fact that about a quarter of patients met the DCPR for type A behavior. According to the DCPR categorical approach, only a limited number of cardiac patients actually display type A behavior. It may thus be important to identify this subgroup, particularly when irritable mood, as in 5 of the 17 patients of that sample, is associated. Two cases met DCPR for illness denial. Even though in this study it does not appear to be a common disturbance, its recognition is worthy of clinical attention. This study therefore underscores the importance of recognizing DCPR syndromes in the CR patient population. The results indicate that half of the patients undergoing CR after an MI present psychological distress which can be subsumed under the DSM or DCPR rubrics. This documents considerable psychosocial needs in this patient population. The findings indicate that DCPR clusters are more suitable for classifying psychological distress in the medically ill than DSM criteria. In particular, in the cited study [14], only 7 of the 61 patients (11%) had a DSM diagnosis, but not a DCPR cluster, whereas 30% of patients could not be identified as presenting psychological distress without the use of DCPR. However, the data lend support to the integration of clinical (DSM) and subclinical (DCPR) criteria for assessing psychological distress in the medically ill [104].

In the other study by Rafanelli et al. [102], 1 month after CABG, at the first psychological assessment during the CR program, 23 of the 47 patients (48.9%) had a DCPR cluster, with a total of 28 DCPR diagnoses. Eight patients (17%) reported type A behavior; 7 (14.9%) irritable mood; 4 (8.5%) health anxiety; 3 (6.4%) demoralization; 2 (4.3%) illness denial; 2 (4.3%) persistent somatization; 1 (2.1%) alexithymia; 1 (2.1%) nosophobia. There was an overlap between the two classification systems. Nine (19.1%) of the 17 patients with DSM-IV diagnoses had an associated DCPR cluster. In 14 cases, therefore, there was a DCPR cluster without any associated psychiatric diagnosis (29.8%). In the cited study, mood disorders were diagnosed in more than 20% of patients. These findings are in accordance with those in the literature [105–114] referring to CABG patients. Differently from those studies, the authors also included the diagnosis of minor depression, as detected in the previous study [14] on MI patients. An important and original result in this investigation concerns the presence of subclinical symptomatology evaluated by DCPR clusters. In almost half of the sample at least one DCPR diagnosis was found with prevalence of type A behavior and irritable mood, as the cardiovascular literature underlined. These data show the importance to include in a clinical assessment both psychiatric (DSM) and subsyndromal psychological states (DCPR), not identified by current nosography, evaluations. The DCPR clusters may have considerable potential for outcome assessment. Further investigations using this assessment methodology in larger patient populations may clarify the role of psychosocial factors in the outcome of CR. Outpatient CR programs offer then an attractive opportunity for systematic screening and intervention for psychosocial problems.

Essential Hypertension

According to Kaplan [115], hypertension presents the largest risk for cardiovascular disease. As blood pressure (BP) increases from normal to severe elevations, the risk for accelerated atherosclerosis, left-ventricular hypertrophy, CHD, and stroke increases markedly [116–119]. Arterial hypertension is defined as a chronic elevation of systolic BP at or above 140 mm Hg, a chronic elevation of diastolic BP at or above 90 mm Hg, or both. In 90% of the people with diagnosed arterial hypertension, the cause for their condition is unknown [120]. Essential hypertension (EH) is the diagnostic label for elevated BP of unknown origins. Because EH is a significant risk factor for morbidity and mortality, the etiology and pathophysiology of EH has been a major focus of biomedical and psychosomatic research for decades [121]. In particular, attempts to link personality factors to the pathophysiology of high BP has been a major area of inquiry and dispute [121–124]. We know that environmental factors play a significant role in the development of EH. High sodium and alcohol intakes and obesity are associated with BP rise with age [125–127]. Physically fit persons have lower incidence of hypertension when compared with less fit persons [128, 129]. Low level of education is related to higher BP [130]. This relation is largely explained by lifestyle factors [130]. On the other hand, cognitive and emotional states can influence BP, heart rate, and vascular perfusion [131]. Past and present theories regarding mechanisms for this potential relationship centre on (a) cardiovascular reactivity to stress, in which a recurrent pattern of exaggerated sympathetic nervous system activity is proposed to upregulate basal BP levels over time; (b) neurohormonal models suggesting that psychological characteristics may predispose hypertension development by altering central nervous system control of baroreceptor function, opioid activity, and neurotransmitter levels, and (c) high-risk behavioral dispositions associated with psychological characteristics, including poor diet, obesity, exercise habits, smoking, and alcohol abuse, among others [132–136]. Psychological factors can raise BP acutely, but whether they affect long-term BP regulation and lead to development of EH, as stated by Alexander [137] at the beginning of the 20th century in his psychosomatic hypothesis, is not known. Over the past decade alone, however, more than 10 longitudinal investigations have released evidence evaluating the effects of psychological factors on hypertension development. The status of psychological factors as a clinically important risk factor for high BP development appears promising, but additional research, potentially including more definite methodological tools in psychosomatic medicine, such as DCPR, will be necessary to further clarify this issue [138].

Psychosocial Antecedents

Acute and Chronic Stress

It is well established that acute stress can lead to a transient increase in BP via changes in cardiac output and vascular resistance [139, 140]. On the other hand, chronic stress can induce prolonged hypertension [141–143]. Hyperreactivity seems to be related to psychosocial aspects. Elevation of BP was associated with unexpected unfortunate life events [136, 144, 145]. In the study by

Osti et al. [144] a consecutive unselected series of 20 outpatients suffering from EH was included. These patients were compared to a control group of 20 patients other than hypertensives, matched for sociodemographic variables. Stressful life events prior to illness onset and psychological distress were investigated. Patients with hypertension were exposed to undesirable life events before disease onset. Evidence about the relationship between these factors and hypertension also points to an autonomic nervous dysfunction [146]. Scarce data are available on the influence of psychological aspects on 24-hour ambulatory BP patterns either in normotensive or hypertensive subjects. A study by Fallo et al. [147] evaluated the relationship between psychological profile and changes in daytime/nighttime BP rhythm. Nocturnal dipping was defined as the night/day ratio of ambulatory mean systolic and/or diastolic BP ≤ 0.87. Three-hundred and two outpatients underwent 24-hour ambulatory BP monitoring. They were administered the Psychosocial Index [148], as an indicator of stress, psychological distress, sleep disturbances, well-being, abnormal illness behavior and quality of life. Patients were divided according to the presence or absence of night BP dipping. Dippers had lower nocturnal systolic and diastolic BP than nondippers, and higher daytime diastolic BP. Patients with nocturnal BP decline had a markedly higher level of stress than nondippers. When the sample was divided according to the presence or absence of hypertension, only subjects with normal BP showed nocturnal dipping associated with increased stressful life circumstances of both acute (e.g. life changes) and chronic (e.g. job strain) nature. The findings lend support to previous investigations linking nighttime BP dipping to an increased number of stressful daily events, and particularly to job strain [149]. The findings suggest the need for 24-hour BP monitoring in patients who are found to be hypertensive during office visits and report life changes and/or stress at work or in the family. Simple questions such as those included in the cited inventory (e.g. 'Did any life changes take place in your life recently? Do you feel under pressure at work? Do you feel tension at home?') may be helpful in this regard. Further research should verify whether stress-reducing techniques may be beneficial in hypertension characterized by BP nighttime dipping. It is conceivable, even though yet to be tested, that psychological approaches aimed at decreasing perception of stress (e.g. cognitive behavioral therapy) or levels of arousal (e.g. relaxation) may be particularly effective [146].

Psychological Aspects

Depression

Recent longitudinal studies [150, 151] have shown a relationship between depression and the subsequent development of hypertension. An increased prevalence of hypertension in depressed patients has been described by Adamis and Ball [152]. They studied the comorbidity between psychiatric and physical diseases in 75 elderly psychiatric inpatients, and found that depressed patients had more cardiovascular diseases and hypertension than other psychiatric patients. Nakagawara et al. [153] also found an increased frequency of hypertension in depressed patients, but only in those with melancholic features. Significantly higher BP was found in 15 subjects with a clinical diagnosis of depression [154]. Prospective studies have also suggested that depression may be a risk factor for the development of hypertension. There is considerable evidence suggesting that hyperreactivity of the sympathetic nervous system and genetic influences are the underlying mechanisms in the relationship between depression and hypertension. Some authors have reported that depression occurred more often in patients with high BP than in those without hypertension [154, 155]; other authors have not confirmed this relationship [156–157]. Clinical studies have reported an association between typical (melancholic) depression and hypertension [150, 154]. Rabkin et al. [154] found a 3-fold higher frequency of major depression in patients treated for hypertension. The physiological mechanisms underlying the relationship between depression and BP probably involve the effect of the sympathetic nervous system.

Although there is no definitive evidence of an association between depression and development of hypertension, depression can impair the management and prognosis of hypertension. On the other hand, hypertension has been proposed as a risk factor for the development of depression. Neuroimaging studies reveal higher frequency of ischemic abnormalities in late-life depression [158]. According to the theory of vascular depression, these abnormalities could represent a vulnerability to depression [152].

Anxiety

Some studies on increased anxiety [159] as a possible psychosomatic mechanism in hypertension suggest that it may have a role in the development of mild high-renin EH. It is well established that anxiety can lead to a transient increase in BP via changes in cardiac output and vascular resistance [139, 140]. Increased risk for hypertension and cardiovascular mortality has been reported in anxiety disorders [161–163]. In the study by Paterniti et al. [131] a stronger relationship between the highest anxiety levels (fourth quartile) and high BP both in men and in women was found. These results could indicate that pathological anxiety is associated with a higher risk of high BP. The strong evidence for an association between high BP and anxiety is supported by a large number of case-control studies that compared either psychological symptoms in hypertensive patients and controls, or BP in patients with a variety of psychiatric disorders and controls [164].

Anger and Hostility

Anger and hostility have long been considered important psychological factors in the development of EH [137, 165–166]. Indeed, Alexander's [137] classic hypothesis, which postulated that chronic inhibition of anger leads to sustained elevations in BP, continues to motivate research in this area nearly seven decades after it was proposed [167, 168]. Although research has identified distinct patterns of cardiovascular activation associated with anger, including increased BP and high peripheral resistance [169, 170], the role of anger in the development and progression of hypertension is still unclear largely because few prospective studies have adequately tested the anger-hypertension hypothesis [171]. Several studies have examined the influence of suppressed hostility or anger ('anger-in') on BP and found that anger-in was positively related to resting BP and/or prevalent hypertension [172], particularly under conditions of stress [173]. However, data from the Framingham study and others do not support this association [174] and some research has found that expressed anger and high levels of trait anger are related to higher BP levels [168, 175]. Moreover, individuals with high levels of expressive hostility or potential for hostility (behavioral measures of hostility associated with both physical and verbal expressions of anger) have shown exaggerated BP responses under conditions of stress or harassment [176, 177] and anger expression has been associated with increased risk of fatal and nonfatal CHD, including MI and angina pectoris [178, 179]. A study by Everson et al. [180] examined the relationship between anger expression and incident hypertension over 4 years in a randomly selected, population-based sample of more than 500 middle-aged men. The data provide strong epidemiological evidence for a positive relationship between anger expression style and subsequent hypertension, independent of known risk factors. Findings support the hypothesis that extreme expression of anger in either direction (anger-in or anger-out, i.e. withholding or repressing feelings and outright displays of anger and aggression) may be related to elevated risk of hypertension. Specific mechanisms by which anger expression increases risk for hypertension remain to be delineated, although the well-documented physiological effects of anger and mental stress make this association biologically plausible. Several lines of evidence indicate that anger and mental stress activate the sympathetic nervous system and hypothalamic-pituitary-adrenal axis, producing increases in heart rate and BP, higher levels of vascular resistance, and secretion of cortisol, catecholamines, glucose, and insulin [169, 170, 181, 182], all of which may contribute to the development or progression of hypertension [183]. Moreover, emerging evidence indicates that local growth factors and endothelial mechanisms, which could be influenced by psychosocial characteristics and stress factors, play an important role in hypertension [183].

Patients with established hypertension have been observed to show greater heart rate and BP increases than normotensive subjects in response to behavioral events such as difficult mental arithmetical operations, or interpersonal interactions designed to arouse fear or anger or to expose personal conflicts [146]. One early study showed that individuals with hypertension reported more restrained aggression and more inner tension than individuals with allergies but without hypertension and hospitalized patients without hypertension [184]. A more recent study comparing participants with borderline hypertension and those with normal BP found that the group with hypertension exhibited less externalized aggression, more internalized aggression, and more submissiveness [160]. However, other studies have failed to detect a relationship between anger or aggression and high BP [185].

Hopelessness

Hopelessness, characterized as a sense of futility and negative expectations about the future and one's personal goals, seems to have cardiovascular consequences that are distinct from or stronger than those associated with depression. The study by Everson et al. [186] examined the relationship between hopelessness and incident hypertension in 616 initially normotensive men, in a 4-year follow-up prospective study in Finland, an area with high rates of cardiovascular disease. Hopelessness was measured by 2 items from a battery of psychosocial questionnaires administered at baseline. These items were 'The future seems to me to be hopeless, and I cannot believe that things are changing for the better' and 'I feel that it is impossible to reach the goals I would like to strive for.' Hopelessness was associated with increased incidence of hypertension. Men reporting high levels of hopelessness at baseline were 3 times more likely to become hypertensive than men who were not hopeless, after adjustments for age, body mass index, baseline resting BP, physical activity, smoking, alcohol consumption, education, parental history of hypertension and self-reported depressive symptoms were taken into consideration [186].

Hypertensive Personality

The 'hypertensive personality' is among the most enduring constructs in psychosomatic medicine. The construct implies that there is an important relationship between psychological variables and the likelihood of developing high BP. A thoughtful review of the literature [123] concluded that although interpretive caution is required, 'a character portrait of the "hypertensive personality" clearly emerges'. This portrait bears a striking resemblance to the descriptions produced by early analytic thinkers [137] and later observers of the personality functioning of hypertensive individuals [184, 187]. That is, hypertensive patients are likely to be characterized by three major factors: (a) their tendency to have conflicts and problems regarding the identification and expression of aggressive feelings; (b) their tendency toward interpersonal isolation, and relative anxiety and strong physiological reactions to interpersonal situations (particularly those that require communication), and (c) their general use of denial, repression, and other inhibiting or distancing defenses to cope with underlying conflicts'. The findings by Friedman et al. [188], however, provide no support for this formulation. The authors' conceptualization of the relationship between psychological characteristics in particular and dispositional variables in general is that they may play a permissive role in the development of hypertension. A more precise understanding of the relationship between personality and elevated BP has been impeded by a number of factors. One concerns psychological theory. No theory about the hypertensive personality is generally accepted, and there is a lack of consensus on which personality or psychological traits are related to BP [188]. A second factor impeding progress toward resolving the hypertensive personality debate is that there is no generally accepted assessment strategy. Hence, several of the studies in the literature did not use standardized psychological tests [185, 188].

Alexithymia

Alexithymia, a concept introduced by Sifneos [189] to describe impoverished fantasy life with a resulting utilitarian way of thinking and a characteristic inability to use appropriate words to describe emotions, has stimulated two decades of psychosomatic research. It has been found that alexithymia is more common in patients with long-lasting psychosomatic conditions than in other subjects. The inhibition of emotional expression and particularly a life-long tendency to suppress anger, have been found to involve increased risk for a variety of health problems both using the alexithymia [189] or similar [190, 191] psychological constructs. Alexithymia is generally considered as a stable personality trait [192–194]. Theories of the causes of alexithymia range from neurobiological to sociocultural ones. Neurobiological theories suggest that alexithymia may be related to an interruption of the limbic-neocortical communication, may be a result of a deficit in interhemispheric communication, or may be a result of a dysfunction in the right cerebral hemisphere [194]. Psychological theories suggest that growing up in an emotionally poor and unstimulating environment or sustaining massive psychological trauma later in life could result in alexithymia [195]. Recently, it has been suggested that alexithymia, regardless of its cause, reflects a deficit in cognitive processing and regulation of emotions [194]. Poor ability to be aware of and to cope with emotions may make an alexithymic individual vulnerable to continuous stress. A recent population study showed that alexithymia is associated with male gender, low educational level, low socioeconomic status, and weakly associated with advanced age [193].

Todarello et al. [196] found a rate of 55% of alexithymia in a group of hypertensive patients in Italy, which contrasted with rates of 33% in a comparison group of Italian psychiatric outpatients and 16% in a community sample. Yula et al. [197] compared newly diagnosed yet untreated, moderately to severely hypertensive subjects with a population sample of men and women of matching age to find out if anger expression, anxiety, hostility, depression, or alexithymia are associated with hypertension. Alexithymia differentiated men and women with untreated hypertension from their normotensive control subjects, whereas anger expression (including suppressed anger) or psychological distress symptoms (including anxiety, depression, and hostility) did not. Alexithymia was associated with elevated BP independent of sodium and alcohol intake, body mass index, and physical fitness. A relatively small portion of the association between BP and alexithymia was mediated by lifestyle factors, mainly by higher relative body weight. Hypertensive and normotensive subjects did not report differences in psychological distress symptoms, which suggests that alexithymia could not be a reaction to the awareness of having elevated BP. Niiranen et al. [198], studied a representative sample of the general adult population (1,440 45- to 74-year-old subjects) in Finland not treated for hypertension. Subjects with sustained hypertension had higher scores in the 20-item Toronto Alexithymia Scale for measuring alexithymia [199, 200] and were thus more alexithymic than those with only clinic hypertension (or 'coat hypertension') and normotensive individuals. Further prospective studies measuring alexithymic personality features, by reliable methods, before elevated BP as well as studies dealing with the neurogenic mechanisms of alexithymia are needed to elucidate its role in the pathogenesis of EH. Self-rating scales, such as the cited Toronto Alexithymia Scale, lack some of the most important pieces of information which can only be obtained by interviews focused on emotions and emotional coping [201]. Yet, they may add further data [5].

Heart Failure

HF is the end stage of many diseases of the heart (ischemic heart disease, hypertensive heart disease, valvular heart disease and cardiomyopathy) and a major cause of morbidity and mortality. Regardless of the severity of the disease, a high level of psychological distress is a significant predictor of hospital readmission [202], poor quality of life [203] and high mortality [204] in cardiac patients. Many findings in patients with CHD are relevant to patients with HF because more than one half of patients with HF have underlying CHD [205], and the two conditions often have shared characteristics. Nonetheless, HF patients have to bear a chronic and life-threatening disease trajectory that is characterized by severe fatigue and dyspnea, deteriorating functional status, episodic adverse cardiac events and repeated hospital readmission [206]. Thus, it is not only physically debilitating, but also psychologically distressing. Moreover, in HF even more than in the case of CHD, the situation is complicated by difficulties in deciding whether to ascribe symptoms like dyspnea, fatigue, insomnia, anorexia, or even palpitation to disease of the heart or of the nervous system [207]. For example depression, when severe enough, can result in malnutrition. Acute mental stress, such as mental arithmetic or a stress interview, can induce transient changes in left ventricular systolic and diastolic function [208] and, in susceptible individuals, the hypertensive and tachycardic reactions are impressive.

Psychological Aspects

Depression

Dickens et al. [209] studied 314 patients admitted to the hospital with a first MI to assess whether HF after MI was predicted by psychosocial characteristics present before the MI. Variables independently associated with worse HF were older age, a history of angina preceding the infarction, and a previous depressive episode (measured by ICD-10 criteria). The impact of depression on postinfarction outcome may result from the influence of preinfarction depression on the degree of cardiac failure.

Studies have shown that patients with HF have high rates of depression compared with the general population. Prevalence rates within studies of HF patients have ranged from 11 to 25% for outpatients and 35 to 70% for inpatients [210]. The wide range of prevalence rates reported across studies is likely the result of the use of different diagnostic instruments and patient populations in terms of mean age, gender makeup and disease severity. The prevalence of depression in CHF patients is similar to rates found in post-MI patients. However it is considerably higher in certain subgroups, such as patients with NYHA class III or IV HF. Depression has been implicated in the progression of CHD as an independent risk factor in both retrospective and prospective studies. Evidence suggests that the presence of depression is independently associated with a poor prognosis for patients with existing HF, in terms of severe functional impairment, mortality and hospital readmission [211], functional decline [204] or death [204, 212, 213]. Moreover, HF patients who are depressed incur health care costs that are 25–40% higher than those who are not depressed, even after controlling for medical comorbidity [214]. In a recent review by MacMahon and Lip [215], it appears that the risk of mortality in patients with HF who are depressed is clearly in need of clinician's attention but is notably lower than the depression associated risk in postinfarction patients. In the study by Fulop et al. [216], the depressed patients with HF used more medical resources after discharge than nondepressed patients. The presence of depression has been shown to decrease adherence to appropriate medical therapy [217, 218].

Anxiety

Existing evidence suggests that the prevalence of anxiety may be as high as 63% depending on the subgroup of HF patients studied [219]. As many as 40% of HF patients may suffer from major anxiety, and overall anxiety levels are 60% higher than levels seen in healthy elders [33]. Compared with other cardiac patients and patients with cancer or lung disease, patients with HF have similarly high or worse anxiety levels [219]. Although anxiety may be an expected and even normal reaction to the diagnosis of a serious chronic illness such as HF, anxiety in patients with cardiac disease is not benign if it persists or is extreme [220–222]. Haworth et al. [223] found that anxiety is common in HF patients living at home: 11% had GAD and 8% PD. One previous small self-report study [224] comprising 50 HF hospitalized participants found a prevalence of 16% for GAD and 12% for PD.

Heart Transplantation

A consistent body of literature has indicated a very high prevalence of psychological disturbances in heart transplant patients [225–228]. These subjects thus offer an excellent opportunity of assessing the performance of different sets of criteria.

DSM Syndromes

The psychiatric evaluation of patients diagnosed with an organic illness such as HF is usually made by using DSM criteria. A study by Grandi et al. [229] aimed to use both DSM-IV criteria and DCPR in a group of outpatients who underwent cardiac transplantation. One hundred and twenty-nine consecutive outpatients were recruited from outpatients attending a Heart Transplantation Unit. All subjects were seen 1 month after the cardiac transplantation. All patients underwent the Italian version of the SCID [230], leading to DSM-IV psychiatric diagnoses. One hundred and six patients (82%) received no DSM psychiatric diagnosis. In the remaining 23 patients, there were 46 DSM diagnoses. As expected, the use of DSM in this setting has confirmed the prevalence on axis I of symptoms related to the anxious/depressive syndromes. GAD and

PTSD were the most frequent diagnostic categories in general and also within the anxiety disorders, followed by specific phobia and agoraphobia. After this group, major depressive episodes and adjustment disorders (with anxious, depressive and irritable mood) were frequent. However, the last diagnostic category is not very useful from a prognostic and therapeutic point of view [231].

DCPR Syndromes

In the cited study by Grandi et al. [229], in all subjects (n = 129) DCPR diagnoses were formulated independently of the DSM-IV diagnostic findings. Only 41 patients out of 129 (31%) received no DCPR diagnosis. In the remaining patients, there were 141 diagnoses. Demoralization, type A behavior, alexithymia and irritable mood were the most frequent diagnostic findings and accounted for roughly 75% of the diagnoses. Also common were health anxiety and illness denial diagnoses.

Feelings of demoralization in heart transplant population seem to be related to the loss of a working position, the reduction of social links and the dependence on other people's support, which creates in the patients a feeling of impotence and loneliness. Patients who were given a DSM diagnosis also presented a DCPR diagnosis. Demoralization was frequently associated with mood disorders and anxiety disorders. As already shown in the literature [232–234], subjects affected by cardiovascular disease seem to present a behavioral pattern characterized by hostility and a sense of being under the pressure of time. The results of the cited study confirm a high prevalence of type A behavior in this sample. Alexithymia accounted for nearly 12% of DCPR diagnoses. The inhibition of emotional expression and particularly a lifelong tendency to suppress anger have been found to involve an increased risk for a variety of health problems, both using alexithymia [189] or similar [190, 191] psychological constructs. Irritable mood appears to be a long-standing syndrome in this population: patients admit to often feeling irritated by someone else's behavior and they declare to make a big effort to contain their anger, which sometimes explodes anyway. It is, however, important to keep in mind that the very stressful circumstances that they have to cope with could exacerbate and amplify an already existent attitude. Health anxiety seemed to be quite common among these patients. Illness denial is reported relatively often in this sample. Mood disorders appear to be related to irritable mood and alexithymia. The overlaps were smaller compared to the previous associations. Anxiety disorders were mostly associated with demoralization, type A behavior and irritable mood [229]. Thirty-seven (28%) of the patients received neither a DCPR diagnosis nor a DSM diagnosis. There were fewer patients (31%) with no DCPR diagnosis than with no DSM-IV diagnosis (82%). Fifty-six patients (43%) who received a DCPR diagnosis were not identified by any DSM-IV diagnosis. Only

3% of patients who received a DSM-IV diagnosis did not receive any DCPR diagnosis. The most frequent associations were between demoralization, type A behavior and irritable mood. The findings of the study by Grandi et al. [229] indicate that diagnostic criteria which may be viewed as encompassing psychosomatic and subclinical variable symptomatology (DCPR) fit better with a medical population than DSM criteria. The number of DCPR diagnoses has been, in fact, almost triple the number of DSM diagnoses. Only a small percentage of patients were not identified by DCPR and this percentage was less than that entailed by DSM criteria. While patients who were given a DSM diagnosis frequently had additional DCPR diagnoses, many patients with DCPR syndromes did not fulfill any DSM criteria. These findings seem to suggest that the DCPR detect psychological dimensions which are not identified by DSM criteria [229]. Finally, the joint use of DSM criteria and DCPR was found to improve the identification of psychological factors in a population of heart transplant patients. Even though it is possible to identify depressive and anxiety symptoms, in the majority of the cases, they are not severe enough to satisfy all the necessary criteria to make a diagnosis. Using DCPR the authors outlined a more specific profile which seems to be characteristic of heart-transplant patients. While the DSM provides important operational tools for identifying and treating mood and anxiety disorders in heart transplant subjects, it fails to provide proper identification, prognostic implications and potential therapeutic implications for this kind of patients in medical practice. There is a pressing need of research in this neglected area. The DCPR provide a step in this direction [229].

Psychological Aspects of Management

Findings that emotional states such as anxiety and depression have a major impact on medical outcomes in cardiac patients suggest that interventions targeting these negative emotions could reduce morbidity and mortality while improving quality of life. Research on the efficacy of interventions for psychological conditions in cardiac patients is quite limited, and much of the literature has been anecdotal, relying heavily on clinical experience and intuition to guide the selection of treatment strategies [25]. The issue of studying and integrating psychosocial interventions into clinical practice would benefit from important measures. The first step in managing cardiac patients should be routine screening to identify those who are severely distressed. Recent data, as strengthened in this article, outline the need to evaluate not only clinical syndromes but also subclinical ones, such as irritable mood, demoralization, illness denial, type A behavior. DCPR could be added in routine screening to better identify specific needs of the patients in cardiac settings. More physicians need thus to be made aware of the recent developments that establish key psychosocial variables as risk factors for the development of CHD and as contributing factors to the expression of disease activity [16]. Secondly, the effectiveness of pharmacological and behavioral interventions for cardiac patients needs to be evaluated in clinical settings. We know that the use of psychotropics in medically ill patients requires attention. These compounds, in fact, may interact with the disease causing several complications. In addition, since the cardiologic patient is often treated with other drugs, the risk of clinically significant pharmacological interactions is obviously improved [235]. Patients with subclinical distress are likely to benefit from CR programs that combine psychosocial interventions with exercise training [236, 237]. There is evidence [238] that CR programs that include psychoeducational components may significantly improve the prognosis of patients recovering from MI. It is conceivable, even though yet to be tested, that programs which are aimed at specific subgroups (e.g. type A behavior, irritable mood, demoralization) may further enhance their effectiveness. In this direction, a proper identification of the psychosocial needs of patients undergoing CR appears to be of primary importance. Psychosocial interventions offered by CR programs can vary widely [239], but interventions such as relaxation training, stress management, psychological support and cognitive restructuring are likely to be beneficial [240]. In particular, the so-called cardiac stress management program is a method, based on principles of behavioral modification, aimed at two objectives: stress management training and change of habitual behavior. Stress management training involves teaching the person how to relax, identify situations inducing stress responses in him or her competitiveness, time pressure, achievement motivation, hostility, and other components of the type A behavior pattern. Other techniques used to treat distress could be incorporated easily into CR programs. For example, scheduling pleasant activities is an important component of some evidence-based interventions for depression [241, 242]. Research indicates that depressed individuals who increase their level of pleasurable activities tend to experience reduced levels of depression [243]. Therefore, in addition to encouraging increased physical exercise, CR clinicians could encourage demoralized patients to become more engaged in pleasurable activities such as reading, visiting friends or gardening. Although comprehensive CR programs that include psychological interventions have been proved effective in reducing subclinical distress [236, 237], these programs are not designed to treat clinical levels of depression. In fact, patients with clinical levels of depression are less likely to gain the full benefit of CR because they tend to drop out of treatment or fail to follow recommendations to reduce cardiac risk factors [243, 244]. This lends support to the importance of treating depression in the setting of MI [44]. Because the problem of lifestyle factors (e.g. smoking, alcohol use) and psychosocial stress frequently cluster together, treatment of patients who are noncompliant with lifestyle changes may benefit from consideration of concomitant psychosocial stresses. Noncompliance may in fact be a sign of anxiety or depression. Patients who report clinically significant levels of anxiety and depression at initial screening should thus be referred to a mental health professional for treatment. Recent studies have assessed the extent to which depression can be successfully treated in cardiac populations. In the SADHART study [245], sertraline was significantly superior to placebo only in the subsets of patients who had a previous depression and those with more severe depression; the incidence of severe cardiovascular adverse events was numerically, but not significantly, greater in the placebo group compared to the sertraline group. Moreover, even though the only randomized behavioral intervention trial (ENRICHD Study) [246] attempting to reduce morbidity and mortality in depressed patients with existing coronary disease showed that changes in depression did not translate into improved survival, there remains the need to further investigate if treating depression can reduce the risk of morbidity and mortality in these patients. As outlined by Rozansky et al. [16], the efficacy of psychosocial interventions may be improved by development of 'patient-specific' treatment plans, based on the 'profiling' of the major psychosocial risk factors in individual patients. In the field of recurrent depression, for example, relapse prevention has been achieved when treatment has been addressed to the individual residual symptoms of patients instead of applying the same approach to all patients [247]. Further studies will confirm if the psychological management of subsyndromal syndromes as well could improve quality of life, through adverse health behaviors, lack of adherence, physical symptom perception, functional impairment and medical utilization. Moreover, there remains the need to further investigate if the management of DCPR syndromes had prognostic implications preventing cardiac morbidity and mortality in these patients.

Conclusions

Using DSM criteria in medical settings, a basic question arises, that is whether patients who do not fulfill these criteria do not indeed present psychological problems which may affect the medical symptoms and are worthy of clinical attention [229]. As outlined in the article, DCPR were alternative diagnostic and conceptual frameworks proposed by an international group of investigators [5]. The findings of the present article indicate that DCPR which may be viewed as encompassing subclinical symptomatology such as irritable mood, demoralization and type A behavior, do fit with a cardiac population and their use might expand the range of a psychological assessment in the setting of cardiovascular disease. There remains the need to further investigate if treating both clinical and subsyndromal psychological conditions can improve quality of life and reduce the risk of morbidity and mortality in these patients. It is clear that further research on the interactions between mental and cardiac health is needed at the clinical, pathophysiological, biochemical and molecular levels if we are to understand the interactions of these two illnesses [248].

References

1 American Psychiatric Association: Diagnostic and Statistical Manual of Mental Disorders, ed 4, Text Revised. Washington, American Psychiatric Press, 2000.

2 Shah SU, White A, White S, Littler WA: Heart and mind. 1. Relationship between cardiovascular and psychiatric conditions. Postgrad Med J 2004;80:683–689.

3 Ketterer MW, Mahr G, Goldberg AD: Psychological factors affecting medical condition: ischemic coronary heart disease. J Psychosom Res 2000;48:357–367.

4 Fava GA, Ruini C, Rafanelli C: Psychometric theory is an obstacle to the progress of clinical research. Psychother Psychosom 2004;73:145–148.

5 Fava GA, Freyberger HJ, Bech P, Christodoulou G, Sensky T, Theorell T, Wise TN: Diagnostic criteria for use in psychosomatic research. Psychother Psychosom 1995;63:1–8.

6 Yusuf S, Hawken S, Ounpuu S, Dans T, Avezum A, Lanas F, McQueen M, Budaj A, Pais P, Varigos J, Lisheng L; INTERHEART Study Investigators: Effect of potentially modifiable risk factors associated with myocardial infarction in 52 countries (the INTERHEART study): case-control study. Lancet 2004;364:937–952.

7 Biondi M, Pancheri P: Fattori psichici che influenzano condizioni mediche; in Pancheri P, Cassano GB (eds): Trattato Italiano di Psichiatria. Milano, Masson, 1999.

8 Libby P, Ridker PM, Maseri A: Inflammation and atherosclerosis. Circulation 2002;105:1135–1143.

9 Reich P: How much does stress contribute to cardiovascular disease? J Cardiovascular Med 1983;8:825–831.

10 Magni G, Corfini A, Berto F, Rizzardo R, Bombardelli S, Miraglia G: Life events and myocardial infarction. Aust N Z J Med 1983;13:257–260.

11 Rafanelli C, Roncuzzi R, Milaneschi Y, Tomba E, Colistro MC, Pancaldi LG, Di Pasquale G: Stressful life events, depression and demoralization as risk factors for acute coronary heart disease. Psychother Psychosom 2005;74:179–184.

12 Paykel ES: The interview for recent life events. Psychol Med 1997;27:301–310.

13 First MB, Spitzer RL, Gibbon M, Williams JBW: SCID-I: Structured Clinical Interview for DSM-IV Axis I Disorders-Patient edition, Biometrics Research Department. New York State Psychiatric Institute, New York (1995) [Italian version: Mazzi F, Morosini P, De Girolamo G, Bussetti M, Guaraldi GP (eds): SCID-I: Intervista Clinica Strutturata per il DSM-IV, i Disturbi dell'asse I. Organizzazioni Speciali OS, Firenze, 2000.

14 Rafanelli C, Roncuzzi R, Finos L, Tossani E, Tomba E, Mangelli L, Urbinati S, Pinelli G, Fava GA: Psychological assessment in cardiac rehabilitation. Psychother Psychosom 2003;72:343–349.

15 Rosengren A, Orth-Gomer K, Wedel H, Wilhelmsen L: Stressful life events, social support, and mortality in men born in 1933. BMJ 1993;307:1102–1105.

16 Rozanski A, Blumenthal JA, Kaplan J: Impact of psychological factors on the pathogenesis of cardiovascular disease and implications for therapy. Circulation 1999;99:2192–2217.

17 Pilowsky I: Abnormal illness behavior. Psychother Psychosom 1986;46:76–84.

18 Wielgosz A, Nolan R, Earp J, Biro E, Wielgosz M: Reasons for patients' delay in response to symptoms of acute myocardial infarction. CMAJ 1988;139:853–857.
19 Levine J, Warrenburg S, Kerns R, Schwartz G, Delaney R, Fontana A, Gradman A, Smith S, Allen S, Cascione R: The role of denial in recovery from coronary heart disease. Psychosom Med 1987;49: 109–117.
20 Julkunen J, Saarinen T: Psychosocial predictors of recovery after a myocardial infarction: development of a comprehensive assessment method. Ir J Psychol 1994;15:67–83.
21 Sirous F: Le deni dans la maladie coronarienne (Denial in coronary artery disease). CMAJ 1992;147:315–321.
22 Lipowski ZJ: Cardiovascular disorders; in Kaplan HI, Freedman AM, Sadock BJ (eds): Comprehensive Textbook of Psychiatry/III. Baltimore/London, Williams & Wilkins, 1980.
23 Goldbeck R: Denial in physical illness. J Psychosom Res 1997;43:573–593.
24 Ottolini F, Modena MG, Rigatelli M: Prodromal symptoms in myocardial infarction. Psychother Psychosom 2005;74:323–327.
25 Doerfler LA, Paraskos JA: Anxiety, posttraumatic stress disorder, and depression in patients with coronary heart disease: a practical review for cardiac rehabilitation professionals. J Cardiopulm Rehabil 2004;24:414–421.
26 Beitman BD, Mukerji V, Lamberti JW: Panic disorder in patients with chest pain and angiographically normal coronary patients arteries. Am J Cardiol 1989;63:1399–1403.
27 Fleet R, Lavoie K, Beitman BD: Is panic disorder associated with coronary artery disease? a critical review of the literature. J Psychosom Res 2000;48:347–356.
28 Jeejeebhoy FM, Dorian P, Newman DM: Panic disorder and the heart: A cardiology perspective. J Psychosom Res 2000;48:393–403.
29 Rutledge T, Reis SE, Olson M, Owens J, Kelsey SF, Pepine CJ, Reichek N, Rogers WJ, Bairey Merz CN, Sopko G, Cornell CE, Sharaf B, Matthews KA: History of anxiety disorders is associated with a decreased likelihood of angiographic coronary artery disease in women with chest pain: The WISE study. J Am Coll Cardiol 2001;37:780–785.
30 Chignon JM, Lepine JP, Ades J: Panic disorder in cardiac outpatients. Am J Psychiatry 1993;150: 780–785.
31 Kubzansky LD, Kawachi I, Weiss ST, Sparrow D: Anxiety and coronary heart disease: a synthesis of epidemiological, psychological, and experimental evidence. Ann Behav Med 1998;20: 47–58.
32 Simon G, Ormel J, VonKorff M, Barlow W: Health care costs associated with depressive and anxiety disorders in primary care. Am J Psychiatry 1995;152:352–357.
33 Denollet J, Brutsaert DL: Personality, disease severity and the risk of long-term cardiac events in patients with a decreased ejection fraction after myocardial infarction. Circulation 1998;97: 167–173.
34 Frasure-Smith N, Lesperance F, Talajic M: Depression and 18-month prognosis after myocardial infarction. Circulation 1995;91:999–1005.
35 Herrmann C, Brand-Driehorst S, Buss U, Ruger U: Effects of anxiety and depression on 5-year mortality in 5,057 patients referred for exercise testing. J Psychosom Res 2000;48:455–462.
36 Moser DK, Dracup K: Is anxiety early after myocardial infarction associated with subsequent ischemic and arrhythmic events? Psychosom Med 1996;58:395–401.
37 Williams RB: Do benzodiazepines have a role in the prevention or treatment of coronary heart disease and other major disorders? J Psychiatr Res 1990;24:51–56.
38 Vingerhoets G: Cognitive, emotional and psychosomatic complaints and their relation to emotional status and personality following cardiac surgery. Br J Health Psychol 1998;3:159–169.
39 Ladwig KH, Schoenfinius A, Dammon G, Danner R, Gurtler R, Hermann R: Long-acting psychotraumatic properties of a cardiac arrest experience. Am J Psychiatry 1999;156:912–919.
40 Doerfler LA: Post-traumatic stress disorder-like symptoms 1 week to 3 months after myocardial infarction. Int J Rehabil Health 1997;3:89–98.
41 Bennett P, Brooke S: Intrusive memories, posttraumatic stress diosrder, and myocardial infarction. Br J Clin Psychol 1999;38:193–199.
42 Doerfler LA, Pbert L, DeCosimo D: Symptoms of posttraumatic stress disorder following myocardial infarction and coronary artery bypass surgery. Gen Hosp Psychiatry 1994;16:193–199.

43 Shemesh E, Rudnick A, Kaluski E, Milovanov O, Salah A, Alon D, Dinur I, Blatt A, Metzkor M, Golik A, Verd Z, Cotter G: Prospective study of posttraumatic stress symptoms and nonadherence in survivors of myocardial infarction. Gen Hosp Psychiatry 2001;23:215–222.
44 Sheps DS, Sheffield D: Depression, anxiety, and the cardiovascular system: the cardiologist's perspective. J Clin Psychiatry 2001;62:12–16.
45 Shemesh E, Yehuda R, Milo O, Dinur I, Rudnick A, Vered Z, Cotter G: Posttraumatic stress, nonadherence, and adverse outcome in survivors of a myocardial infarction. Psychosom Med 2004;66: 521–526.
46 Smith TW, Ruiz JM: Psychosocial influences on the development and course of coronary heart disease: current status and implications for research and practice. J Consult Clin Psychol 2002;70:548–568.
47 Kawachi I, Colditz GA, Ascherio A, Rimm EB, Giovannucci E, Stampfer MJ, Willett WC: Prospective study of phobic anxiety and risk of coronary heart disease in men. Circulation 1994; 89:1992–1997.
48 Littman AB: A review of psychosomatic aspects of cardiovascular disease; in Fava GA, Freyberger H (eds): Handbook of Psychosomatic Medicine. Madison, International Universities press, 1998, pp 261–293.
49 Bush DE, Ziegelstein RC, Patel UV, Thombs BD, Ford DE, Fauerbach JA, McCann UD, Stewaer KJ, Tsilidis KK, Patel AL, Feuerstein CJ, Bass EB: Post-myocardial Infarction Depression. Agency for Healthcare Research and Quality. Rockville, MD, 2005.
50 Freedland KE, Lustman PJ, Carney RM, Hong BA: Underdiagnosis of depression in patients with coronary artery disease: the role of non specific symptoms. Int J Psychiatry Med 1992;22:221–229.
51 Lane D, Carroll D, Ring C, et al: Mortality and quality of life 12 months after myocardial infarction: effects of depression and anxiety. Psychosom Med 2001;63:221–230.
52 Lett HS, Blumenthal JA, Babyak MA, Sherwood A, Strauman T, Robins C, Newman MF: Depression as a risk factor for coronary artery disease: evidence, mechanism and treatment. Psychosom Med 2004;66:305–315.
53 Barth J, Schumacher M, Herrmann-Lingen C: Depression as a risk factor for mortality in patients with coronary heart disease: a meta-analysis. Psychosom Med 2004;66:802–813.
54 Van Melle JP, de Jonge P, Spiijkerman TA, Tijssen JGP, Ormel J, van Veldhuisen DJ, van den Brink RHS, van den Berg MP: Prognostic association of depression following myocardial infarction with mortality and cardiovascular events: a meta-analysis. Psychosom Med 2004;66:814–822.
55 Evans DL, Charney DS, Lewis L, Golden RN, Gorman JM, Krishnan KR, et al: Mood disorders in the medically ill: scientific review and recommendations. Biol Psychiatry 2005;58: 175–189.
56 Borowicz L, Royall R, Grega M, Selnes O, Lyketsos K, McKhann G: Depression and cardiac morbidity 5 years after coronary artery bypass surgery. Psychosomatics 2002;43:464–471.
57 Rafanelli C, Roncuzzi R, Milaneschi Y: Minor depression as a cardiac risk factor after coronary artery bypass surgery. Psychosomatics 2006;47:289–295.
58 Frasure-Smith N, Lesperance F, Talajic M: Depression following myocardial infarction: impact on 6 month survival. JAMA 1993;270:1819–1825.
59 Bunker SJ, Colquhoun DM, Esler MD, Hickie IB, Hunt D, Jelinek VM, Oldenburg BF, Peach HG, Ruth D, Tennant CC, Tonkin AM: 'Stress' and coronary heart disease: psychosocial risk factors. Med J Aust 2003;178:272–276.
60 Lespérance F, Frasure-Smith N, Juneau M, Théroux P: Depression and 1-year prognosis in unstable angina. Arch Intern Med 2000;160:1354–1360.
61 Lesperance F, Frasure-Smith N, Talajic M, Bourassa MG, et al: Five-year risk of cardiac mortality in relation to initial severity and one-year changes in depression symptoms after myocardial infarction. Circulation 2002;105:1049–1053.
62 Carney RM, Freedland KE, Rich MW, et al: Ventricular tachycardia and psychiatric depression in patients with coronary artery disease. Am J Med 1993;95:23–28.
63 Sheps D, Rozansky A: From feeling blue to clinical depression: exploring the pathogenicity of depressive symptoms and their management in cardiac practice. Psychosom Med 2005;67:S2–S5.
64 Carney RM, Freedland KF, Veith RC: Depression, the autonomic nervous system and coronary artery disease. Psychosom Med 2005;67:S29–S33.

65 Bruce FC, Musselman DL: Depression, alterations in platelet function and ischemic heart disease. Psychosom Med 2005;67:S34–S36.
66 Shins A, Honig A, Crijns H, Baur L, Hamulyak K: Increased coronary events in depressed cardiovascular patients: 5-HT2a receptor as missing link? Psychosom Med 2003;65:729–737.
67 Kop WJ, Gottdiener JS: The role of immune system parameters in the relationship between depression and coronary artery disease. Psychosom Med 2005;67:S37–S41.
68 Everson SA, Goldberg DE, Kaplan GA, Cohen RD, Pukkala E, Tuomilehto J, Salonen JT: Hopelessness and risk of mortality and incidence of myocardial infarction and cancer. Psychosom Med 1996;58:113–121.
69 Everson SA, Kaplan GA, Goldberg DE, Salonen JT: Hopelessness and 4-year progression of carothid atherosclerosis: the Kupio ischemic heart disease risk factor study. Arterioscler Thromb Vasc Biol 1997;17:1490–1495.
70 Appels A, Mulder P: Excess fatigue as a precursor of myocardial infarction. Eur Heart J 1988;9: 758–764.
71 Schmale AH, Engel GL: The giving up-given-up complex illustrated on film. Arch Gen Psychiatry 1967;17:135–145.
72 Bech P: Measurement of psychological distress and well-being. Psychother Psychosom 1990;54: 77–89.
73 De Figuereido JM: Depression and demoralization: phenomenological differences and research perspectives. Compr Psychiatry 1993;34:308–311.
74 Fava GA: Screening and diagnosis of depression. Dis Manage Health Outcomes 1997;2:1–7.
75 Fava GA: Irritable mood and physical illness. Stress Med 1987;3:293–299.
76 Mangelli L, Fava GA, Grassi L, Ottolini F, Paolini S, Porcelli P, Rafanelli C, Rigatelli M, Sonino N: Irritable mood in Italian patients with medical disease. J Nerv Ment Dis 2006;194:1–3.
77 Slater E, Roth M: Irritabilità; in Mayer-Gross W (ed): Slater and Roth Clinical Psychiatry. London, Bailliere, Tindall and Cassell, 1969, pp.137–141.
78 Snaith RP, Taylor CM: Irritability. Br J Psychiatry 1985;147:127–136.
79 Fava GA, Grandi S: Differential diagnosis of hypochondriacal fears and beliefs. Psychother Psychosom 1991;55:114–119.
80 Fava GA: The concept of psychosomatic disorder. Psychother Psychosom 1992;58:1–12.
81 Lucock MP, Morley S: The health anxiety questionnaire. Br J Health Psychol 1996;1:137–150.
82 Wells A, Hackmann A: Imagery and core beliefs in health anxiety: content and origins. Behav Cogn Psychother 1993;21:265–273.
83 Johnston DW: The current status of the coronary prone behaviour pattern. J R Soc Med 1993;86: 406–409.
84 Friedman M, Rosenman RH: Association of a specific overt behaviour pattern with increases in blood cholesterol: blood clotting time: incidence of arcus senilis and clinical coronary artery disease. JAMA 1959;169:1286–1296.
85 Rosenman RH, Friedman M, Strauss R, Wurm M, Kositchek R, Hahn W, et al: A predictive study of coronary heart disease. JAMA 1964;189:15–22.
86 Friedman M, Powell LH: The diagnosis and quantitative assessment of Type A behaviour. Integr Psychiatry 1984;2:123–129.
87 Littman AB: Review of psychosomatic aspects of cardiovascular disease. Psychother Psychosom 1993;60:148–167.
88 Haynes SG, Feinleib M, Kannel WB: The relationship of psychosocial factors to coronary heart disease in the Framingham study: 3. Eight year incidence of coronary heart disease. Am J Epidemiol 1980;111:37–58.
89 Rosenman RH, Brand RJ, Sholtz RI, Friedman M: Multivariate prediction of coronary heart disease during 8.5 year follow-up in Western Collaborative Group Study. Am J Cardiol 1976;37: 903–909.
90 Shekelle RB, Hulley SB, Neaton JD, Billings J, Borhani NO, Gerace TA, Jacobs DR, Lasser NL, Mittlemark MB, Stamler J: The MRFIT behavior pattern study. II. Type A behavior and incidence of coronary heart disease. Am J Epidemiol 1985;122:559–570.
91 Johnston DW, Cook DG, Shaper AG: Type A behaviour and ischaemic heart disease in middle aged British men. BMJ 1987;295:86–89.

92 Hearn M, Murray DM, Luepker RB: Hostility, coronary heart disease and total mortality: a 33 year follow up study of university students. J Behav Med 1989;12:105–121.
93 Nunes EV, Frank KA, Kornfield DS: Psychologic treatment for the type A behaviour pattern for coronary heart disease: a meta-analysis of the literature. Psychosom Med 1987;48:159–173.
94 Oldridge NB, Giyatt GH, Fisher ME, Rinn AA: Cardiac rehabilitation after myocardial infarction. Combined experience of randomised clinical trials. JAMA 1988;260:945–950.
95 O'Connor GT, Buring JE, Yusuf S, Goldhaber SZ, Olmstead EM, Paffenbarger RS, Hennekens CH: An overview of randomized trials of rehabilitation with exercise after myocardial infarction. Circulation 1989;80:234–244.
96 Donker FJS: Cardiac rehabilitation: a review of current developments. Clin Psychol Rev 2000;220: 923–943.
97 Grace SL, Abbey SE, Shnek ZM, Irvine J, Franche RL, Stewart DE: Cardiac rehabilitation I: review of psychosocial factors. Gen Hosp Psychiatry 2002;24:121–126.
98 Grace SL, Abbey S, Shnek Z, Irvine J, Franche RL, Stewart D: Cardiac rehabilitation. 2. Referral and participation. Gen Hosp Psychiatry 2002;24:127–134.
99 First, MB, Spitzer RL, Gibbon M, Williams JBW: Structured Clinical Interview for DSM IV Axis I Disorders (SCID-I) Biometrics Research Department. New York, New York State Psychiatric Institute, 1994.
100 American Psychiatric Association: Diagnostic and Statistical Manual of Mental Disorders, ed 4. Washington, DC, APA Press, 1994.
101 Lavic C, Dilani R, Cassidy M, Gilliland Y: Effects of cardiac rehabilitation and exercise training programs in women with depression. Am J Cardiol 1999;83:1480–1483.
102 Rafanelli C, Roncuzzi R, Milaneschi Y: Minor depression as cardiac risk factor after coronary artery by-pass surgery. Psychosomatics 2006;47:289–295.
103 Freyberger HJ: Interview for field trials of Diagnostic Criteria for Psychosomatic Research (DCPR). Lubeck, University of Lubeck, 1995.
104 Fava GA, Mangelli L, Ruini C: Assessment of psychological distress in the setting of medical disease. Psychother Psychosom 2001;70:171–175.
105 Burker EJ, Blumenthal JA, Feldman M, Burnett R, White W, Smith LR, Croughwell N, Schell R, Newman M, Reves JG: Depression in male and female patients undergoing cardiac surgery. Br J Clin Psychol 1995;34:119–128.
106 Pirraglia PA, Peterson JC, Williams-Russo P, Gorkin L, Charlson ME: Depressive symptomatology in coronary artery bypass graft surgery patients. Int J Geriatr Psychiatry 1999;14:668–680.
107 Underwood MJ, Firmin RK, Jehu D: Aspects of psychological and social morbidity in patients awaiting coronary artery bypass grafting. Br Heart J 1993;69:382–384.
108 McKhann GM, Borowicz LM, Goldsborough MA, Enger C, Selnes OA: Depression and cognitive decline after coronary artery bypass grafting. Lancet 1997;349:1282–1284.
109 Burg MM, Benedetto MC, Rosenberg R, Soufer R: Presurgical depression predicts medical morbidity 6 months after coronary artery bypass graft surgery. Psychosom Med 2003;65:111–118.
110 Timberlake N, Klinger L, Smith P, Venn G, Treasure T, Harrison M, Newman SP: Incidence and patterns of depression following coronary artery bypass graft surgery. J Psychosom Res 1997;43: 197–207.
111 Saur CD, Granger BB, Muhlbaier LH, Forman LM, McKenzie R, Taylor MC, Smith PK: Depressive symptoms and outcome of coronary artery bypass grafting. Am J Crit Care 2001;10: 4–10.
112 Baker RA, Andrew MJ, Schrader G, Knight JL: Preoperative depression and mortality in coronary artery bypass surgery: preliminary findings. ANZ J Surg 2001;7:139–142.
113 Connerney I, Shapiro PA, McLaughlin JS, Bagiella E, Sloan RP: Relation between depression after coronary artery bypass surgery and 12-month outcome: a prospective study. Lancet 2001;358:1766–1771.
114 Blumenthal JA, Lett HS, Babyak MA, White W, Smith PK, Mark DB, Jones R, Mathew JP, Newman MF and NORG Investigators: Depression as a risk factor for mortality after coronary artery bypass surgery. Lancet 2003;362:604–609.
115 Kaplan NM: Importance of coronary heart disease risk factors in the management of hypertension: an overview. Am J Med 1989;86:1–4.

116 Castelli W: Epidemiology of coronary heart disease. Am J Med 1984;76:4–12.
117 Frohlich ED, Apstein C, Chobanian AV, Devereux RB, Dustan HP, Fauad-Tarazi F, Horan MJ, Marcus M, Massie B, Pfefer MA, Re RN, Roccella EJ, Savage D, Shub C: The heart in hypertension. N Engl J Med 1992;327:998–1008.
118 Kaplan NM: Clinical Hypertension, ed 5. Baltimore, Williams & Wilkins, 1990.
119 Sambhi MP, Chobanian AV, Julius S, Noth RH, Borhani NO, Perry HM: University of California, Davis, Conference: Mild hypertension. Am J Med 1988;85:675–696.
120 Guyton AC: Textbook of Medical Physiology, ed 6. Philadelphia, W. B. Saunders, 1981.
121 Johnson EH, Gentry WD, Julius S (eds): Personality, Elevated Blood Pressure, and Essential Hypertension. Washington, DC, Hemisphere, 1992.
122 Linden W: Psychological Perspectives of Essential Hypertension: Etiology, Maintenance, and Treatment. Basel, Switzerland, Karger, 1984.
123 Sommers-Flanagan J, Greenberg RP: Psychosocial variables and hypertension: a new look at an old controversy. J Nerv Mental Dis 1989;177:15–24.
124 Suls J, Wan CK, Costa PT: Relationship of trait anger to resting blood pressure: a meta-analysis. Health Psychol 1995;14:444–456.
125 Intersalt Cooperative Research Group. Intersalt: an international study of electrolyte and blood pressure: results for 24 hour urinary sodium and potassium excretion. BMJ 1988;297: 319–328.
126 Elliott P, Stamler J, Nichols R, Dyer AR, Stamler R, Kesteloot H, Marmot M; for the Intersalt Cooperative Research Group. Intersalt revisited: further analyses of 24 hour sodium excretion and blood pressure within and across populations. BMJ 1996;312:1249–1253.
127 Marmot MG, Elliott P, Shipley MJ, Dyer AR, Ueshima H, Beevers DG, Stamler R, Kesteloot H, Rose G, Stamler J: Alcohol and blood pressure: the Intersalt study. BMJ 1994;308: 1263–1267.
128 Paffenbarger RS, Wing AL, Hyde RT, Jung DL: Physical activity and incidence of hypertension in college alumni. Am J Epidemiol 1983;117:245–257.
129 Blair SN, Goodyear NN, Gibbons LW, Cooper KH: Physical fitness and incidence of hypertension in healthy normotensive men and women. JAMA 1984;252:487–490.
130 Stamler R, Shipley M, Elliott P, Dyer A, Sans S, Stamler J: Higher blood pressure in adults with less education: some explanations from Intersalt. Hypertension 1992;19:237–241.
131 Paterniti S, Alpérovitch A, Ducimetière P, Dealberto MJ, Lépine JP, Bisserbe JC: Anxiety but not depression is associated with elevated blood pressure in a community group of French elderly. Psychosom Med 1999;61:77–83.
132 Pickering TG, Gerin W: Cardiovascular reactivity in the laboratory and the role of behavioral factors in hypertension: a critical review. Ann Behav Med 1990;12:3–16.
133 Matthews KA, Woodall KL, Allen MT: Cardiovascular reactivity to stress predicts future blood pressure status. Hypertension 1993;22:479–485.
134 Kaplan JR, Pettersson K, Manuck SB, Olsson G: Role of sympathoadrenal medullary activation in the initiation and progression of atherosclerosis. Circulation 1991;84:23–32.
135 Krantz DS, Manuck SB: Acute psychophysiological reactivity and the risk of cardiovascular disease: a review and methodological critique. Psychol Bull 1984;96:435–464.
136 James SA: Psychosocial precursors of hypertension: a review of the epidemiologic evidence. Circulation 1987;76:60–66.
137 Alexander F: Emotional factors in essential hypertension. Psychosom Med 1939;1:175–179.
138 Rutledge T, Hogan BE: A quantitative review of prospective evidence linking psychological factors with hypertension development. Psychosom Med 2002;64:758–766.
139 Whitehead WE, Blackwell B, De Silva H, Robinson A: Anxiety and anger in hypertension. J Psychosom Res 1994;21:383–389.
140 Shapiro D, Goldstein IB, Jamner LD: Effects of cynical hostility, anger out, and defensiveness on ambulatory blood pressure in black and white college students. Psychosom Med 1996;58:354–364.
141 Forsyth RP, Hoffbrand BI, Melmon KL: Hemodynamic effects of angiotensin in normal and environmentally-stressed monkeys. Circulation 1971;44:119–126.
142 Jonsonn A, Hanson L: Prolonged exposure to a stressful stimulus (noise) as a cause of raised blood pressure in man. Lancet 1977;1:86–87.

143 Cobb S, Rose RM: Hypertension, peptic ulcer and diabetes in air traffic controllers. JAMA 1973;224:489–492.
144 Osti RM, Trombini G, Magnani B: Stress and distress in essential hypertension. Psychother Psychosom 1980;33:193–197.
145 Buck CW, Donner AP: Blood pressure control in hypertensives – a model for the study of life events. J Chronic Dis 1984;37:247–253.
146 Light KC: Psychosocial precursors of hypertension: experimental evidence. Circulation 1987;76: 67–76.
147 Fallo F, Barzon L, Rabbia F, Navarrini C, Conterno A, Veglio F, Cazzaro M, Fava GA, Sonino N: Circadian blood pressure patterns and life stress. Psychother Psychosom 2002;71:350–356.
148 Sonino N, Fava GA: A simple instrument for assessing stress in clinical practice. Postgrad Med J 1998;74:408–410.
149 Theorell T, de Faire U, Johnson J, Hall E, Perski A, Stewart W: Job strain and ambulatory blood pressure profiles. Scand J Work Environ Health 1991;17:380–385.
150 Jonas BS, Franks P, Ingram DD: Are symptoms of anxiety and depression risk factors for hypertension? Longitudinal evidence from the National Health and Nutrition Examination Survey I Epidemiologic Follow-up Study. Arch Fam Med 1997;6:43–49.
151 Simonsick EM, Wallace RB, Blazer DG, Berkman LF: Depressive symptomatology and hypertension-associated morbidity and mortality in older adults. Psychosom Med 1995;57:427–435.
152 Adamis D, Ball C: Physical morbidity in elderly psychiatric inpatients: prevalence and possible relations between the major mental disorders and physical illness. Int J Geriatr Psychiatry 2000;15: 248–253.
153 Nakagawara M, Witzke W, Matussek N: Hypertension in depression. Psychol Res 1987;21:85–86.
154 Rabkin JG, Charles E, Kass F: Hypertension and DSM-III depression in psychiatric outpatients. Am J Psychiatry 1983;140:1072–1074.
155 Wells KB, Golding JM, Burnam A: Affective, substance use, and anxiety disorders in persons with arthritis, diabetes, heart disease, high blood pressure, or chronic lung conditions. Gen Hosp Psychiatry 1989;11:320–327.
156 Wheatley D, Balter M, Levine J, Lipman R, Bauer ML, Bonato R: Psychiatric aspects of hypertension. Br J Psychiatry 1975;127:327–336.
157 Friedman MJ, Bennet PL: Depression and hypertension. Psychosom Med 1977;39:134–142.
158 Greenwald BS, Kramer-Ginsberg E, Krishnan KR, Hu J, Ashtari M, Wu H, Aupperle P, Patel M, Pollack S: A controlled study of MRI signal hyperintensities in older depressed patients with and without hypertension. J Am Geriatr Soc 2001;49:1218–1225.
159 Thailer SA, Friedman R, Harshfield GA, Pickering TG: Psychologic differences between high-, normal-, and low-renin hypertensives. Psychosom Med 1985;47:294–297.
160 Perini C, Muller FB, Buhler FR: Suppressed aggression accelerates early development of essential hypertension. J Hypertens 1991;9:499–503.
161 Noyes R, Clancy J, Hoenk TR, Slymen DJ: The prognosis of anxiety neurosis. Arch Gen Psychiatry 1980;37:173–176.
162 Coryell W, Noyes R, House JD: Mortality among outpatients with anxiety disorders. Am J Psychiatry 1986;143:508–512.
163 Fontaine R, Boisvert D: Psychophysiological disorders in anxious patients: hypertension and hypotension. Psychother Psychosom 1982;38:165–172.
164 Pilgrim GA: Psychological aspects of high and low blood pressure. Psychol Med 1994;24:9–14.
165 Ayman D: The personality type of patients with arteriolar essential hypertension. Am J Med Sci 1933;186:213–223.
166 Diamond EL: The role of anger and hostility in essential hypertension and coronary heart disease. Psychol Bull 1982;92:410–433.
167 Markowitz JH, Matthews KA, Wing RR, Kuller LH, Meilahn EN: Psychological, health behavior and biological predictors of blood pressure change in middle-aged women. J Hypertens 1991;9:399–406.
168 Harburg E, Gleiberman L, Russell M, Cooper ML: Anger coping styles and blood pressure in blacks and whites. Psychosom Med 1991;53:153–164.
169 Schwartz GE, Weinberger DA, Singer JA: Cardiovascular differentiation of happiness, sorrow, anger, and fear following imagery and exercise. Psychosom Med 1981;43:343–367.

170 Sinha R, Lovallo WR, Parsons OA: Cardiovascular differentiation of emotions. Psychosom Med 1992;54:422–435.
171 Suls J, Wan C, Costa PT: Relationship of trait anger to resting blood pressure: a meta-analysis. Health Psychol 1995;14:444–456.
172 Goldstein HS, Edelberg R, Meier CF, Davis L: Relationship of resting blood pressure and heart rate to experienced anger and expressed anger. Psychosom Med 1988;50:321–329.
173 Cottington EM, Matthews KA, Talbott E, Kuller LH: Occupational stress, suppressed anger, and hypertension. Psychosom Med 1986;48:249–260.
174 Haynes SG, Levine S, Scotch N, Feinleib M, Kannel WB: The relationship of psychosocial factors to coronary heart disease in the Framingham study. Am J Epidemiol 1978;107:362–383.
175 Laude D, Girard A, Consoli S, Mounier-Vehier C, Elghozi JL: Anger expression and cardiovascular reactivity to mental stress: a spectral analysis approach. Clin Exp Hypertens 1997;19: 901–911.
176 Everson SA, McKey BS, Lovallo WR: Effect of trait hostility on cardiovascular responses to harassment in young men. Intl J Behav Med 1995;2:172–191.
177 Miller SB, Dolgoy L, Friese M, Sita A: Dimensions of hostility and cardiovascular response to interpersonal stress. J Psychosom Res 1996;41:81–95.
178 Mittleman MA, Lewis RA, Maclure M, Sherwood JB, Muller JE: Triggering of acute myocardial infarction onset by episodes of anger. Circulation 1995;92:1720–1725.
179 Kawachi I, Sparrow D, Spiro A, Vokonas P, Weiss ST: A prospective study of anger and coronary heart disease. The Normative Aging Study. Circulation 1996;94:2090–2095.
180 Everson SA, Goldberg DE, Kaplan GA, Julkunen J, Salonen J: Anger expression and incident hypertension. Psychosom Med 1998;60:730–735.
181 Muller JE, Tofler GH, Stone PH: Circadian variation and triggers of onset of acute cardiovascular disease. Circulation 1989;79:733–743.
182 Vitaliano PP, Scanlan JM, Krenz C, Fujtmoto W: Insulin and glucose: relationships with hassles, anger, and hostility in nondiabetic older adults. Psychosom Med 1996;58:489–499.
183 Kaplan NM: Clinical Hypertension, ed 7. Baltimore, Williams & Wilkins, 1998, pp 41–99.
184 Wolf S, Wolff HG: A summary of experimental evidence relating life stress to the pathogenesis of essential hypertension in man; in Bell ET (ed): Hypertension. Minneapolis, University of Minnesota Press, 1951, pp 457–491.
185 Sparrow D, Garvey AJ, Rosner B, Thomas HE: Factors in predicting blood pressure change. Circulation 1982;65:789–794.
186 Everson SA, Kaplan GA, Goldberg DE, Salonen JT: Hypertension incidence is predicted by high levels of hopelessness in Finnish men. Hypertension 2000;35:561–567.
187 Saslow G, Gressel GC, Shobe FO, DuBois PH, Schroeder HA: Possible etiologic relevance of personality factors in arterial hypertension. Psychosom Med 1950;12:292–302.
188 Friedman R, Schwartz J, Schnall PL, Landbergis PA, Pieper C, Gerin W, Pickering TG: Psychological variables in hypertension: relationship to casual or ambulatory blood pressure in men. Psychosom Med 2001;63:19–31.
189 Sifneos PE: The prevalence of 'alexithymic' characteristics in psychosomatic patients. Psychother Psychosom 1973;22:255–262.
190 Greer J: Cancer and the mind. Br J Psychiatry 1983;143:535–543.
191 Berry DS, Pennebaker JW: Nonverbal and verbal emotional expression and health. Psychother Psychosom 1993;59:11–19.
192 Kauhanen J, Julkunen J, Salonen JT: Validity and reliability of the Toronto Alexithymia Scale (TAS) in a population study. J Psychosom Res 1992;36:687–694.
193 Salminen JK, Saarijarvi S, Toikka T, Kauhanen J: Prevalence of alexithymia and its association with sociodemographic variables in the general population of Finland. J Psychosom Res 1999;46: 75–82.
194 Taylor GJ, Bagby RM, Parker JDA: Disorders of Affect Regulation: Alexithymia in Medical and Psychiatric Illness. Cambridge, UK, Cambridge University Press, 1997.
195 Krystal H: Integration and Self-Healing: Affect, Trauma, Alexithymia. Hillsdale, NJ, Analytic Press, 1988.
196 Todarello O, Taylor GJ, Parker JDA, Fanelli M: Alexithymia in essential hypertension and psychiatric outpatients: a comparative study. J Psychosom Res 1995;39:987–994.

197 Yula A, Salminen J, Saarijarvi S: Alexithymia: a facet of essential hypertension. Am Heart J 1999;33:1057–1061.
198 Niiranen TJ, Jula AM, Kantola IM, Reunanen A: Prevalence and determinants of isolated clinic hypertension in the Finnish population: the Finn-HOME study. J Hypertension 2006;24:463–470.
199 Bagby RM, Parker JD, Taylor GJ: The Twenty-item Toronto Alexithymia Scale – I. Item selection and cross-validation of the factor structure. J Psychosom Res 1994;38:23–32.
200 Bagby RM, Taylor GJ, Parker JD: The Twenty-item Toronto Alexithymia Scale – II. Convergent, discriminant, and concurrent validity. J Psychosom Res 1994;38:33–40.
201 Sifneos PE: Affect, emotional conflict and deficit. An overview. Psychother Psychosom 1991;56: 116–122.
202 Levine JB, Covaino NA, Slack VW, et al: Psychological predictors of subsequent medical care among patients hospitalized with cardiac disease. J Cardiopulm Rehabil 1996;16:109–116.
203 Lane D, Carroll D, Ring C, Beevers DG, Lip GYH: Mortality and quality of life 12 months after myocardial infarction. Psychosom Med 2001;63:221–230.
204 Vaccarino V, Kasl SV, Abramson J, Krumholz HM: Depressive symptoms and risk of functional decline and death in patients with heart failure. J Am Coll Cardiol 2001;38:199–205.
205 Kannel WB, Ho K, Thom T: Changing epidemiological features of cardiac failure. Br Heart J 1994;72:S3–S9.
206 Yu DS, Lee DT, Woo J, Thompson DR: Correlates of psychological distress in elderly patients with congestive heart failure. J Psychosom Res 2004;57:573–581.
207 Skotzko CE, Krichten C, Zietowski G, Alves L, Freudenberger R, Robinson S, Fisher M, Gottlieb SS: Depression is common and precludes accurate assessment of functional status in elderly patients with congestive heart failure. J Card Fail 2000;6:300–305.
208 Giannuzzi P, Shabetai R, Imparato A, Temporelli PL, Bhargava V, Cremo R, Tavazzi L: Effects of mental exercise in patients with dilated cardiomyopathy and congestive heart failure: an echocardiographic Doppler Study. Circulation 1991;83:155–165.
209 Dickens C, Percival C, Tomenson B, Heagerty A: Association between depressive episode before first myocardial infarction and worse cardiac failure following infarction. Psychosomatics 2005;46:523–528.
210 Joynt KE, Whellan DJ, O' Connor CM: Why is depression bad for the failing heart? A review of the mechanistic relationship between depression and heart failure. J Card Heart Fail 2004;10: 258–271.
211 Jiang W, Alexander J, Christopher J, Kuchibhatla M, Gaulden LH, Cuffe MS, Blazing MA, Davenport C, Califf RM, Krishnan RR, O'Connor CM: Relationship of depression to increased risk of mortality and rehospitalization in patients with congestive heart failure. Arch Int Med 2001;161:1849–1856.
212 Murberg TA, Bru E, Svebak S, Tveteras R, Aarsland T: Depressed mood and subjective health symptoms as predictors of mortality in patients with congestive heart failure: a two-years follow-up study. Int J Psychiatry Med 1999;29:311–326.
213 Faris R, Purcell H, Henein MY, Coats AJ: Clinical depression is common and significantly associated with reduced survival in patients with non-ischaemic heart failure. Eur J Heart Fail 2002; 4:541–551.
214 Frasure-Smith N, Lesperance F, Gravel G, et al: Depression and health care costs during the first year following myocardial infarction. J Psychosom Res 2000;48:471–478.
215 MacMahon KM, Lip GY: Psychological factors in heart failure: a review of the literature. Arch Int Med 2002;162:509–516.
216 Fulop G, Strain JJ, Stettin G: Congestive heart failure and depression in older adults: clinical course and health services use 6 month after hospitalization. Psychosomatics 2003;44: 367–373.
217 Koenig HG: Depression in hospitalized older patients with congestive heart failure. Gen Hosp Psychiatry 1998;20:29–43.
218 Carney RM, Freedland KE, Eisen SA, et al: Major depression and medication adherence on coronary artery disease. Health Psychol 1995;14:88–90.
219 De Jong MJ, Moser DK, An K, Chung ML: Anxiety is not manifested by elevated heart rate and blood pressure in acutely ill cardiac patients. Eur J Cardiovasc Nurs 2004;3:247–253.

220 Januzzi JL, Stern TA, Pasternak RC, DeSantis RW: The influence of anxiety and depression on outcomes of patients with coronary artery disease. Arch Intern Med 2000;160:1913–1921.
221 Kubzansky LD, Kawachi I: Gooing to the heart of the matter: do negative emotions cause coronary heart disease? J Psychosom Res 2000;48:323–327.
222 Mayou RA, Gill D, Thompson DR, Day A, Hicks N, Volmink J, et al: Depression and anxiety as predictors of outcome after myocardial infarction: effects of depression and anxiety. Psychosom Med 2000;62:212–219.
223 Haworth JE, Moniz-Cook E, Clark AL, Wang M, Waddington R, Cleland JGF. Prevalence and predictors of anxiety and depression in a sample of chronic heart failure patients with left ventricular systolic dysfunction. Eur J Heart Fail 2005;7:803–808.
224 Griez EJL, Mammar N, Loirat JC, Djega N, Trochut JN, Bouhour JB: Panic disorder and idiopatic cardiomyopathy. J Psychosom Res 2000;48:585–587.
225 Goldman LS, Kimball CP: Psychiatric aspects of cardiac surgery: a review. Cardiovasc Rev Rep 1985;3:1023–1034.
226 Schroeder JS: Current status of cardiac transplantation. JAMA 1997;241:2069–2071.
227 Stukas AA Jr, Dew MA, Switzer GE, DiMartini A, Kormos RL, Griffith BP: PTSD in heart transplant recipients and their primary family caregivers. Psychosomatics 1999;40:212–221.
228 Dew MA, DiMartini AF, Switzer GE, Kormos RL, Schulberg HC, Roth LH, Griffith BP: Patterns and predictors of risk for depressive and anxiety-related disorders during the first three years after heart transplantation. Psychosomatics 2000;41:191–192.
229 Grandi S, Fabbri S, Tossani E, Mangelli L, Branzi A, Magelli C: Psychological evaluation after cardiac transplantation: the integration of different criteria. Psychother Psychosom 2001;70:176–183.
230 Spitzer RL, Williams JBW, Gibbon M, First MB: Structured Clinical Interview for DSM-III-R, Version 1.0 (SCID). American Psychiatric Press, Washington, DC, 1990. (Italian version: Fava M, Guaraldi GP, Mazzi F, Rigatelli M (eds). SCID-I Intervista Clinica Strutturata per il DSMIII-R Organizzazioni Speciali OS, Firenze, 1993.
231 Grassi L, Mangelli L, Fava GA, Grandi S, Ottolini F, Porcelli P, Rafanelli C, Rigatelli M, Sonino N: Psychosomatic characterization of adjustment disorders in the medical setting: some suggestions for DSM-V. J Affect Disord 2006, Dec 27.
232 Littman AB: Review of psychosomatic aspects of cardiovascular disease. Psychother Psychosom 1993;60:148–167.
233 Rosenman RH, Brand RJ, Jenkins CD, Friedman M, Straus R, Wurm M: Coronary heart disease in Western Collaborative Group Study: Final follow-up experience of 8 and a half years. JAMA 1975;233:872–877.
234 Coelho R, Ramos E, Prata J, Barros H: Psychosocial indexes and cardiovascular risk factors in a community sample. Psychother Psychosom 2000;69:261–274.
235 Fasullo S, Puccio D, Fasullo S, Novo S: La terapia farmacologica della depressione dopo infarto miocardico acuto. Ital Heart J Suppl 2004;5:839–846.
236 Linden W, Stossel C, Maurice J: Psychosocial interventions for patients with coronary artery disease. Arch Intern Med 1996;156:745–752.
237 World Health Organization: Needs and Action Priorities in Cardiac Rehabilitation and Secondary Prevention in Patients with Coronary Heart Disease. Geneva, WHO Regional Office for Europe, 1993.
238 Dusseldorp E, van Elderen T, Maes S, Meulman J, Kraaij V: A meta-analysis of psychoeducational programs for coronary heart disease. Health Psychol 1999;18:506–519.
239 Barlow DH: Anxiety and Its Disorders, ed 2. New York, Guilford, 2002.
240 Nathan PE, Gorman JM (eds): A Guide to Treatments That Work, ed 2. New York, Oxford, 2002.
241 Beck AT, Rush AJ, Shaw BF, Emery G: Cognitive Therapy of Depression. New York, Guiford, 1979.
242 Levinsohn PM, Gotlib IH: Behavioral theory and treatment of depression; in Beckam EE, Leber WR (eds): Handbook of Depression, ed 2. New York, Guilford, 1995, pp 352–375.
243 Lane D, Carroll D, Ring C, Beevers DG, Lip GYH: Predictors of attendance at cardiac rehabilitation after myocardial infarction. J Psychosom Res 2001;51:497–501.
244 Ziegelstein RC, Fauerbach JA, Stevens SS, Romanelli J, Richter DP, Bush DE: Patients with depression are less likely to follow recommendations to reduce cardiac risk during recovery from a myocardial infarction. Arch Intern Med 2000;160:1818–1823.

245 Glassman AH, O'Connor CM, Califf RM, et al; for the SADHART (Sertraline Anti-Depressant Heart Attack Randomised Trial) Group: Sertraline treatment of major depression in patients with acute MI or unstable angina. JAMA 2002;288:701–709.
246 ENRICHD investigators: Enhancing recovery in coronary heart disease patients (ENRICHD): study design and methods. Am Heart J 2000;139:1–9.
247 Fava GA: Long-term treatment with antidepressant drugs. Psychother Psychosom 2002;71: 127–132.
248 Shabetai R: Depression and heart failure. Psychosom Med 2002;64:13–14.

Chiara Rafanelli, MD, PhD
Department of Psychology, University of Bologna
Viale Berti Pichat, 5
IT–40127 Bologna (Italy)
Tel. +39 051 2091847, Fax +39 051 243086, E-Mail chiara.rafanelli@unibo.it

Porcelli P, Sonino N (eds): Psychological Factors Affecting Medical Conditions. A New Classification for DSM-V. Adv Psychosom Med. Basel, Karger, 2007, vol 28, pp 109–126

Toward a Biopsychosocial Approach to Skin Diseases

Angelo Picardi[a], *Paolo Pasquini*[b]

[a]Italian National Institute of Health, Centre of Epidemiology, Surveillance and Health Promotion, [b]Dermatological Institute IDI-IRCCS, Rome, Italy

Abstract

A link between the mind and the skin has long been hypothesized. Indeed, some studies suggested that psychosocial factors may play a role in the pathogenesis and course of several skin diseases. Conversely, other studies suggested that psychiatric disorders and psychosocial difficulties may result as a complication of a primary skin disease. Epidemiological studies indeed found a high prevalence of psychiatric disorders among dermatological patients. This is a source of concern, because psychiatric morbidity is associated with emotional suffering, disability, lower quality of life, poorer adherence to dermatological treatment, and increased risk of self-harm. Conditions such as demoralization, health anxiety, irritable mood, type A behavior, and alexithymia were also found to be frequent in dermatological patients, and to be independently associated with greater psychological distress, lower quality of life, and poorer psychosocial functioning. Several studies also raised concerns about underrecognition and undertreatment of psychiatric disorders. This large body of findings suggests that psychosocial issues deserve more attention in everyday dermatological practice, and highlights the need for a biopsychosocial approach to the management of patients with skin disease. To this purpose, the development of efficient consultation-liaison services enabling an effective collaboration between dermatologists and mental health professionals is mandatory.

Skin diseases are quite frequent. For instance, the prevalence of psoriasis alone in the general population has been estimated between 0.6 and 4.8% [1], and population-based studies in Europe yielded estimates of 2–3% [2].

These diseases can present with many different symptoms, including pain, itching, burning, stinging, blistering, thickening, alterations in skin pigmentation or skin color, and hair or eyebrow loss. The lesions may be visible and may cause cosmetic damage or disfigurement.

Dermatological diseases may carry a substantial burden on those affected, and their influence on patients' lives may be quite destructive. Several patients report experiences of stigmatization [3], and many of them complain of restricted daily activities and impaired quality of life [4].

Psychological Antecedents

The Link between the Mind and the Skin

The skin has substantial psychological implications and is tightly linked to the brain and the mind. It plays a key role as a sensory organ in socialization processes, is responsive to various emotional stimuli, and affects an individual's body image and self-esteem. Also, the skin and the central nervous system are embryologically related, because both the epidermis and the neural plate derive from the embryonic ectoderm. Moreover, the skin and the central nervous system share many hormones, neurotransmitters, and receptors [5].

Therefore, it is not surprising that the possibility of a causal influence of psychological factors, particularly emotional stress, on the course of various skin diseases has long been postulated.

The Role of Stressful Events in Skin Diseases

While many anecdotal observations and uncontrolled case-series support the common opinion that stressful life events can precipitate the onset or recurrence of many skin diseases, the picture emerging from controlled studies is less straightforward.

The role of stressful life events in triggering or exacerbating lichen planus, pemphigus and seborrheic dermatitis is either controversial or insufficiently explored. Their role in psoriasis, alopecia areata, atopic dermatitis, acne, urticaria, and vitiligo is supported by some studies, although only a few of them met acceptable methodological standards for stress measurement, and no study controlled for the influence of possible confounding factors such as discontinuation of ongoing medical treatment, alcohol, smoking, exposure to sunlight, or seasonal effects [6].

The Role of Social Support and Individual Difference Factors

In a recent series of studies [7–10], we found no or only weak evidence of an association between stressful events and the onset of alopecia areata or the exacerbation of psoriasis and vitiligo. Rather, these studies suggested that a key role in modulating susceptibility to skin disease may be played by poor social support and by individual difference factors related to emotion regulation, such as alexithymia and insecure attachment.

The presence of high alexithymic characteristics, as measured by the 20-item Toronto Alexithymia Scale, increased the risk of experiencing an exacerbation of plaque psoriasis and vitiligo, and tended to increase the risk of developing alopecia areata.

Insecure attachment, particularly attachment-related avoidance, was also found to increase vulnerability to skin disease. High attachment-related avoidance tended to increase the risk of developing alopecia areata; also, higher attachment-related avoidance was associated with a recent exacerbation of plaque psoriasis and tended to be associated with a recent exacerbation of vitiligo. Further, high attachment-related anxiety was found to increase the risk of experiencing an exacerbation of vitiligo.

Moreover, lower perceived social support was found to be associated with a recent exacerbation of plaque psoriasis and vitiligo, and tended to be associated with the onset of alopecia areata.

In contrast, no association was found between the onset or exacerbation of alopecia areata, plaque psoriasis, and vitiligo and either the total number of recent (last 12 months) stressful life events or the number of undesirable, uncontrollable, and major events. The only exception was the finding of an association between the exposure to three or more uncontrollable events and the exacerbation of vitiligo.

These findings are consistent with the large body of literature documenting that good social relationships are associated with health, and that social support is a protective factor for health [11, 12]. Interestingly, a recent population-based study corroborated an association between poor social support and increased skin morbidity [13]. The importance of social support as a buffering factor in dermatological patients has been highlighted also by the recent finding that psychological distress is associated more strongly with poor social support than with clinical status and physical symptoms of itching in patients with psoriasis and atopic dermatitis [14].

Our findings also suggest that individual difference factors may play a cardinal role, possibly greater than that of stressful events themselves, in increasing the vulnerability to skin disease. Indeed, stress theories emphasize that stress is inherent neither to the environment nor the person alone, but results from their interplay [15]. Stressful events and situations do not impact on an inert object. Models postulating that causality flows from stress as a stimulus to the stress reaction as an outcome are overly simplistic. An individual's emotions, thoughts, and behaviors contribute to the onset and maintenance of stress.

Individual difference factors influence the stress process in many aspects as they can affect the descriptive situation representations, the appraisal of stress situations, and the coping processes. They are also crucial in the selection and shaping of stress situations [16]. Indeed, a role of individual differences is also suggested by some studies reporting that some dermatological patients seem to be 'stress reactors', while others are not [17–19].

Alexithymia is characterized by reduced ability to identify and verbally express emotions, limited symbolic thinking, and poor fantasy life. Individuals high in alexithymia have impaired emotion regulation, and they may inaccurately perceive subjective stress states in the presence of stressful events or situations and thus may be less able to cope with the stressors. Some psychophysiological studies indeed suggested that alexithymia may bias the perception of stress and lead to a decoupling between subjective and physiological responses to stress [20].

Interestingly, a recent Turkish study on patients with alopecia areata corroborated a possible role of alexithymia, while no association with stressful life events was found [21]. Another recent study suggested a link between lower ability to integrate and differentiate emotions and reactivity to stress among patients with psoriasis [22].

Attachment insecurity may affect stress regulation in that it may increase perceived stress, may affect the intensity or duration of the physiological stress response, and may determine the success of social support in buffering stress as it is associated with lower propensity to seek partner support and ineffective support seeking. Evidence linking attachment insecurity not only with mental but also with physical health has started to accumulate [23]. Recently, high attachment-related avoidance was found to be associated with poorer natural killer cell cytotoxicity, independently of perceived stress and social support [24].

Our finding of an association between insecure attachment and susceptibility to skin disease are consistent with those of a previous pilot study, performed on an heterogeneous sample of patients with various skin diseases [25]. Although insecure attachment may also result in elevated use of external regulators of affect such as smoking or drinking, in our studies the association between insecure attachment and skin disease onset or exacerbation was independent from alcohol or tobacco use.

Research is also starting to reveal interesting relationships between attachment style and subjective quality of life in dermatological patients [26].

Possible Physiological Mediators

Several physiological mechanisms may mediate the interplay between stress, individual difference factors, and skin disease. Research is gradually uncovering a complex neuroendocrine-immune network that may reasonably account for a mind-body connection in the skin [27].

In vulnerable individuals, stress-induced release of neuroimmune substances may adversely affect cutaneous homeostasis through activation of inflammatory processes in deeper skin layers [28]. A recent study revealed an interesting correlation between low salivary cortisol ratios, a marker of chronic stress, and an increased number of substance P- and neurokinin-1 receptor-positive inflammatory cells in the skin of patients with psoriasis [29]. Also, psychological stress has been shown to alter epidermal permeability barrier, which may facilitate the development or the persistence of inflammatory skin diseases [30]. Furthermore, stress has been shown to compromise the skin wound-healing response [31].

Psychiatric and Psychological Aspects

Prevalence of Psychiatric Disorders among Dermatological Patients

Psychiatric disorders are frequent among patients with skin diseases [32]. In a large epidemiological study on 2,579 dermatological outpatients, we found a prevalence of psychiatric morbidity, as measured by the 12-item General Health Questionnaire (GHQ-12), of 25% [33]. In another large study on 545 dermatological inpatients, the prevalence of psychiatric morbidity, as determined with the Structured Clinical Interview for DSM-IV Disorders Axis I, was as high as 38%. The more frequent disorders were mood (20%) and anxiety (16%) disorders, the most common diagnoses being major depressive disorder (7%), generalized anxiety disorder (6%), dysthymic disorder (5%), and panic disorder (4%). Adjustment disorders and somatoform disorders were also frequent, with a prevalence of 7% for both diagnostic categories [34]. Visibility of lesions seems to increase the risk of psychiatric morbidity [35–37], especially among female patients [37].

Our finding of a high prevalence of psychiatric morbidity among dermatological patients is consistent with previous studies on diagnostically heterogeneous patient samples carried out in a variety of nations [35, 38–43]. Several other studies on patients with specific diseases such as psoriasis, acne, atopic dermatitis, alopecia areata, urticaria, vitiligo, and pruritus, highlighted the frequent presence of psychiatric morbidity [22, 44–52].

The Issue of Suicidal Ideation

A particularly alarming finding concerns the high prevalence of suicidal ideation among patients with skin diseases. Recently, we administered the Patient Health Questionnaire (PHQ), a self-report instrument yielding DSM-IV diagnoses, to 466 dermatological patients (309 outpatients and 177 inpatients). The PHQ explicitly and specifically enquires about suicidal ideation: 'over the last two weeks, how often have you been bothered by thoughts that you would be better off dead or of hurting yourself in some way?'. A percentage as high as 8.6% of patients reported the presence of suicidal ideation. In 3% of patients, suicidal thoughts were experienced more than half of days or nearly all days. Even considering only outpatients, the prevalence of suicidal ideation was still 4.8%.

The validity of the assessment of suicidal ideation is supported by the fact that it was absent in 58 patients with minor skin problems (nevi, mycosis, cheratosis, warts). In contrast, it was frequent among patients with acne (7.1%), skin tumors (8.3%), various dermatitides (8.8%), psoriasis (10%), and urticaria (18.8%) [53].

This finding is in line with previous reports of frequent suicidal ideation and even cases of completed suicide among dermatological patients. In a study of 480 patients with psoriasis, mild-to-moderate facial acne, atopic dermatitis, or alopecia areata who completed the Carroll Rating Scale for Depression, suicidal ideation and death wishes were present among 4 and 7.3% of patients, respectively [48]. In another study, suicidal ideation as measured by the relevant item of the Beck Depression Inventory was quite common among patients with psoriasis (21%) and atopic dermatitis (19%) [54]. A Pakistani study found a prevalence of suicidal ideation of 8% among acne patients [55].

Furthermore, some patients with acne scars have been reported to have become suicidal even after successful dermabrasion [56]. Also, several cases of dermatological patients who completed suicide have been reported [57]. In a survey of 341 consultant dermatologists in the UK, participants reported that they knew of 178 and 28 patients who had either attempted or completed suicide, respectively [58].

Correlates of Psychiatric Morbidity

The presence of psychiatric morbidity in dermatological patients has several important correlates. First, it is associated with impaired health-related quality of life [59] and, interestingly, this association is not limited to the social or psychological domains of quality of life. In a study on 2,136 dermatological outpatients, for all symptomatic skin conditions the presence of psychiatric morbidity as determined by the GHQ-12 was associated with greater burden of skin symptoms on quality of life [60].

This finding is consistent with those of other studies which suggested a link between emotional state and severity of itch and other cutaneous sensory symptoms [61–63]. Indeed, being stressed was found to be associated with severity of various cutaneous sensory symptoms even in nonclinical subjects [64].

Second, psychiatric morbidity is associated with poorer adherence to dermatological treatment. In a longitudinal study of 396 first-visit outpatients, a strong association was found between psychiatric morbidity and poor adherence to the dermatologist's prescriptions. The risk of poor adherence was increased about three times in patients with psychiatric comorbidity as compared with patients free from psychiatric comorbidity [65].

Prevalence of Diagnostic Criteria for Psychosomatic Research Conditions among Dermatological Patients

In the aforementioned study on dermatological inpatients [34], we found that the classical psychiatric diagnostic criteria alone may not provide a full description of psychological distress conditions in patients with skin diseases, and may be profitably supplemented by the Diagnostic Criteria for Psychosomatic Research (DCPR) which are particularly suitable for identifying psychological distress in medically ill patients.

While 38% of participants received a DSM-IV diagnosis, a percentage as high as 48% of them received a DCPR diagnosis. Overall, 13% received only a DSM-IV diagnosis, 25% received both a DSM-IV and a DCPR diagnosis, while 22.8% received only a DCPR diagnosis.

Patients diagnosed with a DCPR condition had most frequently an overlapped DSM-IV diagnosis of depressive (28.3%) and anxiety (26%) disorders, whereas patients with a DSM-IV disorder had substantial overlap with demoralization (30.1%), functional somatic symptoms secondary to a psychiatric disorder (23.8%), irritable mood (18.0%), and type A behavior (15.0%).

It is worth noting that almost half (47.7%) of patients with a DCPR condition did not have an overlapped DSM-IV diagnosis [66] and as such would have not been detected as patients with mental health needs, had the DCPR not been used.

The most frequent DCPR diagnoses were demoralization, functional somatic symptoms secondary to a psychiatric disorder (both 14.1%), irritable mood (13.7%), type A behavior (12%), health anxiety (10.6%), and alexithymia (5.9%). Table 1 reports the prevalence estimates for all DCPR conditions.

The high prevalence of demoralization is not surprising, given the profound link between the skin, body image, and self-esteem. The frequent occurrence of irritable mood is consistent with many investigations highlighting the frequent presence of irritability and anger in a variety of skin diseases, such as acne [67, 68], psoriasis [69], and atopic dermatitis [70]. While type A behavior has been extensively researched in patients with cardiovascular disease, our findings suggest that it can also be commonly observed among other patient populations.

Abnormal illness behavior is an important focus of attention of DCPR. Health anxiety was quite prevalent in our sample, and this finding is consistent with previous studies indicating that it relates to high concern of acute illness signs and is frequent among subjects who are referred to medical services for their health status [71]. However, the number of patients with other DCPR conditions characterized by abnormal illness behavior, such as disease phobia, persistent somatization, thanatophobia, conversion symptoms, and illness denial, was not negligible, being around 2% for each of these conditions.

Table 1. Prevalence of DCPR conditions among dermatological inpatients (n = 539)

DCPR diagnosis	Patients	Prevalence (95% CI)
Demoralization	76	14.1 (11.3–17.3)
Functional somatic symptoms secondary to a psychiatric disorder	76	14.1 (11.3–17.3)
Irritable mood	74	13.7 (10.9–16.9)
Type A behaviour	65	12.0 (9.4–15.1)
Health anxiety	57	10.6 (8.1–13.5)
Alexithymia	32	5.9 (4.1–8.3)
Disease phobia	12	2.2 (1.2–3.9)
Thanatophobia	12	2.2 (1.2–3.9)
Conversion symptoms	12	2.2 (1.2–3.9)
Persistent somatization	11	2.0 (1.0–3.6)
Illness denial	10	1.8 (0.9–3.4)
Anniversary reaction	7	1.3 (0.5–2.6)
Any DCPR diagnosis	258	47.9 (43.6–52.2)
Only one DCPR diagnosis	140	26.0 (22.3–29.9)
Two or more DCPR diagnoses	118	21.9 (18.5–25.6)
Only DCPR without DSM diagnoses	123	22.8 (19.3–26.6)
Both DCPR and DSM-IV diagnoses	135	25.0 (21.4–28.9)

The common presence of mood, irritable, and anxious conditions among patients with skin disease may also favor the appearance of secondary, functional somatic symptoms through a vicious circle of selective perception and disease interpretation of somatic sensations [72].

The presence of either a DSM-IV psychiatric diagnosis or a DCPR condition was associated not only with increased levels of psychological distress as measured by the GHQ-12, but also with higher impairment of quality of life in the functioning and emotions domains as measured by the Skindex-29 questionnaire. It is of particular importance that the presence of a DCPR condition, but not of a DSM-IV diagnosis, was associated also with higher impairment in quality of life related to symptoms of skin disease [34].

Alexithymic features, particularly difficulty identifying feelings, were also found to be associated with reduced global psychosocial functioning, independently of psychiatric comorbidity or burden of skin symptoms [73].

Besides DCPR conditions, other individual difference factors such as attachment security, which has already been commented upon, and dispositional social sensitivity, which was found to be associated with poorer social functioning and quality of life among patients with acne [74], are also worth of clinical attention.

Psychosocial Implications for the Management of Skin Diseases

The Complex Relationship between Dermatological and Psychosocial Morbidity

The relationship between psychiatric and dermatological morbidity is complex. Most studies in the field have a simple cross-sectional design which is not suitable for investigating causal relationships. However, some case-control studies on patients with various skin diseases [7–10, 21, 25, 75–79], a small prospective study on patients with psoriasis [80], a prospective study on patients with atopic dermatitis [81], and a recent prospective study on students with acne undergoing examination stress [82] did suggest a causal role for psychosocial factors in several skin diseases.

On the other hand, a longitudinal study found an increased risk of developing psychiatric morbidity in patients with skin disease who do not improve with dermatological treatment [83]. This finding corroborates several elegant studies on patients with skin diseases which highlighted the relevance of experiences of stigmatization [84–87] and illness-related stress [88, 89], and their correlation with emotional distress and psychosocial disability. Hence, the available evidence suggests that the link between psychiatric and dermatological morbidity is, likely, bidirectional.

The Recognition of Psychiatric Disorders in Dermatological Patients

Independently from the direction of the association between psychosocial and dermatological morbidity, the high prevalence of psychiatric disorders and psychological conditions of psychosomatic relevance among patients with skin disease should be taken into serious consideration, as it is associated with emotional suffering, impaired quality of life, poorer adherence to dermatological treatment, worse outcome, and even risk of self-harm.

Several excellent papers have been published to guide the assessment of psychopathology in the dermatological patient [5, 90, 91]. This issue is of more than academic importance, because for most dermatological patients with comorbid psychiatric or psychological conditions it will take long before they see a mental health professional. Hence, dermatologists have a key role in early detection and treatment.

On the positive side, dermatologists are probably even better than psychiatrists in recognizing the presence of psychopathology in certain patients, namely those suffering from a psychiatric disorder that presents as a dermatological complain. The rare Ekbom's syndrome or delusion of parasitosis is a classic example. The patient has a delusional disorder characterized by the firm belief of being infested with parasites despite clear evidence to the contrary, while psychosocial functioning in most areas of life is preserved. Such patients often resist psychiatric referral, and the dermatologist has a major role in treatment.

Self-inflicted skin lesions are a more common problem and can be found in a broad spectrum of psychiatric disorders. While the patient is often under psychiatric treatment, sometimes the dermatologist is the first to see the patient and has an important role in differential diagnosis and referral to mental health specialists. Self-inflicted lesions are produced through repetitive scratching, typically do not conform to those of known dermatoses, and are grouped at easily accessible and usually exposed sites of the body, such as the extensor surfaces of the extremities, face and upper back. The lesions are usually of similar size and shape, they often exhibit delayed healing due to recurrent picking, and they are characterized as clean, linear erosions, scabs and scars that are frequently hypopigmented or hyperpigmented.

Usually the patient acknowledges the self-inflicted nature of the lesions; in this case, the old-fashioned diagnostic label 'neurotic excoriations' is often used. If the patient negates the self-inflicted nature of the lesions and denies emotional distress, the condition is labeled as 'dermatitis artefacta' [92]. This disorder is difficult to treat and should be differentiated from clear malingering.

Trichotillomania is a particular case of self-inflicted skin mutilation that involves hair pulling. The scalp is the more frequently involved site. The clinical presentation of the lesions is usually characteristic: hairs at the occiput and base of the head are spared, resulting in a tonsural pattern of baldness. Patches have irregular borders and contain hairs of varying length, the shortest being those most recently removed. However, in some cases histology may be needed for a correct diagnosis [93].

On a less positive side, dermatologists seem to be less able to recognize mental health issues among patients with a 'normal' skin disease. The available evidence suggests that psychiatric and psychological morbidity goes often unrecognized among such patients.

In a recent study on 46 dermatologists (82% of all dermatologists working in a dermatological hospital), we tested the correspondence between dermatologists' opinions and the actual data collected in a large epidemiological study carried out in the same institution a few months before. In patients affected by some classical skin diseases, such as psoriasis, vitiligo, alopecia, lichen planus, pruritus, acne, and urticaria, we observed a good concordance between dermatologists' opinions and epidemiological data. However, there was a substantial underestimation of concurrent psychiatric morbidity in patients with other skin diseases, such as contact dermatitis, herpes zoster infections, bacterial infections, insect bites, herpes simplex infections, warts, and nail diseases [94].

Possibly, dermatologists referred mainly to the clinical severity of the various skin conditions in order to form their opinions about the frequency of depressive or anxiety disorders in each condition. This would explain why they underestimated the prevalence of anxiety and depression in several relatively mild conditions. However, there is no straightforward relationship between the clinical severity of the skin condition and psychological adjustment. Many psychosocial factors may account for the large individual variation in adjustment [95], and it has been found that the impact of skin disease on quality of life is more strongly associated with psychiatric morbidity than the clinical severity of the disorder [33].

Even less encouraging were the findings of another recent study on 277 dermatological outpatients, which directly assessed the dermatologists' ability to recognize depressive and anxiety disorders in their patients. The dermatologists identified the presence of mental health problems in only 13 of 39 (33%) patients with a psychiatric disorder as measured by the PHQ. In most cases of disagreement between the dermatologists and the PHQ, the GHQ-12 corroborated the PHQ classification [96].

Although limitations inherent in self-report psychiatric assessment should be considered, this study suggests that mental disorders often go unrecognized in dermatological patients, and its results are consistent with those of other studies which found that psychiatric disorders go frequently undetected in everyday dermatological clinical practice [38, 97].

Steps towards Improving the Recognition of Psychiatric Morbidity

Surely, busy clinical routines and limited time do not help dermatologists to address the mental health needs of their patients. To this purpose, several steps may be undertaken.

Educational programs for dermatologists might be implemented to increase their skills in diagnosing and managing mental disorders. The effectiveness of such programs has been documented in general practitioners [98]. Clearly, such programs should not aim at turning dermatologists into psychiatrists, but rather at helping them to recognize emotional distress and feeling more comfortable in dealing with psychiatric and psychological issues [99].

Also, self-administered questionnaires to screen for general psychiatric morbidity, such as the GHQ-12, or to screen specifically for depressive disorders, such as the PHQ or the Primary Care Screener for Affective Disorders, have been validated in dermatological patients [100–102] and may help clinicians to identify patients with concurrent psychiatric morbidity.

However, neither educational nor screening programs by themselves are likely to bring substantial improvement in patient outcomes. In primary care, simple guideline implementation strategies and educational strategies were found to have limited effectiveness in changing clinical practice and improving the outcome of psychiatric disorders [103].

Also, an emphasis on increased recognition alone is probably insufficient to change patient outcomes, particularly in settings lacking systems to assure accurate diagnosis, effective treatment, and careful follow-up [104, 105]. While dermatologists have a key role in identifying patients with comorbid psychiatric or psychological conditions, they also need support from mental health professionals in order to manage these patients most effectively. Unfortunately, such support is not always available, and several dermatologists complain about the scarce availability of local clinical psychology or psychiatric liaison services [58].

Therefore, educational and screening programs aimed at increasing recognition of psychiatric disorders should be supplemented by the development of efficient consultation-liaison services [106] and the implementation of quality improvement programs [107], in order to provide effective treatment and careful follow-up of dermatological patients with mental health needs. Given that mental health services and the professionals working in them are often hard-pressed, promoting liaison work may be difficult initially, but things tend to get better once contacts are opened and maintained [108].

The Need for a Biopsychosocial Approach to Skin Diseases

Research findings consistently attest to the importance of addressing psychological and social factors in the management of skin diseases, because such factors may affect the course and the prognosis of skin conditions.

For instance, psychological distress was found to be associated with increased time to clearance of psoriasis in patients receiving photochemotherapy [109]. Conversely, cognitive-behavioral stress management techniques delivered in group format were found to have a beneficial impact on psoriasis clinical severity [110]; also, a meditation-based stress reduction approach reduced time to clearance of psoriasis in patients treated with phototherapy or photochemotherapy [111].

The limitations inherent in a strictly medical approach to skin diseases with complex effects on patients' daily experience, such as psoriasis, were recently underscored by the finding that while clearance of lesions produces a significant reduction in psoriasis-related disability, it does not impact upon emotional distress or coping [112].

The potential benefits of the integration of mental health interventions into standard care protocols are further suggested by the finding of clinical improvement in most patients referred to a liaison psychiatrist within a dermatology clinic [113].

All these results corroborate the view that many skin conditions should be considered in the context of biopsychosocial factors [114]. Building up a fruitful, mutual collaboration between dermatologists and mental health professionals in the framework of a shared biopsychosocial approach is an important step towards improving patient outcomes.

Conclusions

A large body of literature has been devoted to the fascinating link between the mind and the skin. On the one hand, psychosocial factors are likely to play a role in the pathogenesis and course of several skin diseases; on the other hand, psychological distress and psychiatric disorders may result as a complication or a consequence of a primary skin disease, in reaction to disfigurement, perceived social stigma, or undesirable lifestyle changes.

As a matter of fact, a high prevalence of psychiatric disorders among patients with skin diseases was found in many studies. This is a source of concern, because psychiatric morbidity causes substantial suffering and is associated with greater impairment in quality of life, poorer medication adherence, increased risk of self-harm and, possibly, worse treatment response and outcome. Although the dermatologists' awareness of the problem is rising, psychiatric disorders still seem to go often unrecognized and are believed to be less frequent than they actually are in many skin conditions.

Several DCPR conditions, such as demoralization, functional somatic symptoms secondary to a psychiatric disorder, irritable mood, type A behavior, health anxiety, and alexithymia, were also found to be very frequent among dermatological patients. The presence of a DCPR condition has substantial clinical relevance as it was found to be independently associated with emotional distress, impaired psychosocial functioning, and greater burden of symptoms of skin disease on quality of life.

These research findings suggest that psychosocial issues are an integral part of skin disease which deserves more attention in everyday clinical practice, and highlight the need for a biopsychosocial approach to patients with skin disease. Conceivably, the identification and treatment of comorbid psychiatric disorders and psychological conditions of psychosomatic relevance may favorably affect the course of skin disease. To this purpose, psychiatric diagnostic criteria may be profitably complemented by the DCPR.

Such a comprehensive assessment of psychological distress in patients with skin diseases, coupled with the development of efficient consultation-liaison services enabling an effective collaboration between dermatologists and mental health professionals in the framework of a shared biopsychosocial approach, should greatly help reaching the ultimate aim of improving patient outcomes.

References

1 Naldi L: Epidemiology of psoriasis. Curr Drug Targets Inflamm Allergy 2004;3:121–128.
2 Schafer T: Epidemiology of psoriasis. Review and the German perspective. Dermatology 2006;212: 327–337.

3 Kent G: Stigmatisation and skin conditions; in Walker C, Papadopoulos L (eds): Psychodermatology. Cambridge, Cambridge University Press, 2005.
4 Bingefors K, Lindberg M, Isacson D: Self-reported dermatological problems and use of prescribed topical drugs correlate with decreased quality of life: an epidemiological survey. Br J Dermatol 2002;147:285–290.
5 Koblenzer CS: Psychosomatic concepts in dermatology. Arch Dermatol 1983;119:501–512.
6 Picardi A, Abeni D: Stressful life events and skin diseases: disentangling evidence from myth. Psychother Psychosom 2001;70:118–136.
7 Picardi A, Pasquini P, Cattaruzza MS, Gaetano P, Baliva G, Melchi CF, Tiago A, Camaioni D, Abeni D, Biondi M: Only limited support for a role of psychosomatic factors in psoriasis: results from a case-control study. J Psychosom Res 2003;55:189–196.
8 Picardi A, Pasquini P, Cattaruzza MS, Gaetano P, Melchi CF, Baliva G, Camaioni D, Tiago A, Abeni D, Biondi M: Stressful life events, social support, attachment security, and alexythimia in vitiligo: a case-control study. Psychother Psychosom 2003;72:150–158.
9 Picardi A, Pasquini P, Cattaruzza MS, Gaetano P, Baliva G, Melchi CF, Papi M, Camaioni D, Tiago A, Gobello T, Biondi M: Psychosomatic factors in first-onset alopecia areata. Psychosomatics 2003;44:374–381.
10 Picardi A, Mazzotti E, Gaetano P, Cattaruzza MS, Baliva G, Melchi CF, Biondi M, Pasquini P: Stress, social support, emotional regulation and exacerbation of diffuse plaque psoriasis. Psychosomatics 2005;46:556–564.
11 Cohen S, Gottlieb BH, Underwood LG: Social relationships and health; in Cohen S, Underwood LG, Gottlieb BH (eds): Social Support Measurement and Intervention: A Guide for Health and Social Scientists. New York, Oxford University Press, 2000.
12 Cacioppo JT, Hawkley LC: Social isolation and health, with an emphasis on underlying mechanisms. Perspect Biol Med 2003;46(suppl 3):S39–S52.
13 Dalgard F, Svensson Å, Sundby J, Dalgard OS: Self-reported skin morbidity and mental health. A population survey among adults in a Norwegian city. Br J Dermatol 2005;153:145–149.
14 Evers AWM, Lu Y, Duller P, van der Valk PGM, Kraaimaat FW, van de Kerkhof PCM: Common burden of chronic skin diseases? Contributors to psychological distress in adults with psoriasis and atopic dermatitis. Br J Dermatol 2005;152:1275–1281.
15 Lazarus RS, Folkman S: Stress, Appraisal, and Coping. Springer, New York, 1984.
16 Vollrath M: Personality and stress. Scand J Psychol 2001;42:335–347.
17 Gupta MA, Gupta AK, Kirkby S, Schork NJ, Gorr SK, Ellis CN, Voorhees JJ: A psychocutaneous profile of psoriasis patients who are stress reactors. A study of 127 patients. Gen Hosp Psychiatry 1989;11:166–173.
18 Niemeier V, Nippesen M, Kupfer J, Schill WB, Gieler U: Psychological factors associated with hand dermatoses: which subgroup needs additional psychological care? Br J Dermatol 2002;146: 1031–1037.
19 Zachariae R, Zachariae H, Blomqvist K, Davidsson S, Molin L, Mork C, Sigurgeirsson B: Self-reported stress reactivity and psoriasis-related stress of Nordic psoriasis sufferers. J Eur Acad Dermatol Venereol 2004;18:27–36.
20 Stone LA, Nielson KA: Intact physiological response to arousal with impaired emotional recognition in alexithymia. Psychother Psychosom 2001;70:92–102.
21 Yazici AC, Basterzi A, Acar ST, Ustunsoy D, Ikizoglu G, Demirseren D, Kanik A: Alopecia areata and alexithymia. Turk Psikiyatri Dergisi 2006;17:101–106.
22 Consoli SM, Rolhion S, Martin C, Ruel K, Cambazard F, Pellet J, Misery L: Low levels of emotional awareness predict a better response to dermatological treatment in patients with psoriasis. Dermatology 2006;212:128–136.
23 Maunder RG, Hunter JJ: Attachment and psychosomatic medicine: developmental contributions to stress and disease. Psychosom Med 2001;63:556–567.
24 Picardi A, Battisti F, Tarsitani L, Baldassari M, Copertaro A, Mocchegiani E, Biondi M: Attachment security and immunity in healthy women. Psychosom Med 2007;69:40–46.
25 Russiello F, Arciero G, Decaminada F, Corona R, Ferrigno L, Fucci M, Pasquini M, Pasquini P: Stress, attachment and skin disease: a case-control study. J Eur Acad Dermatol Venereol 1995;5: 234–239.

26 Schmidt S: Female alopecia: the mediating effect of attachment patterns on changes in subjective health indicators. Br J Dermatol 2003;148:1205–1211.
27 Tausk FA, Nousari H: Stress and the skin. Arch Dermatol 2001;137:78–82.
28 Panconesi E, Hautmann G: Psychophysiology of stress in dermatology. The psychobiologic pattern of psychosomatics. Dermatol Clin 1996;14:399–421.
29 Remrod C, Lonne-Rahm S, Nordlind K: Study of substance P and its receptor neurokinin-1 in psoriasis and their relation to chronic stress and pruritus. Arch Dermatol Res 2007;299:85–91.
30 Garg A, Chren MM, Sands LP, Matsui MS, Marenus KD, Feingold KR, Elias PM: Psychological stress perturbs epidermal permeability barrier homeostasis: implications for the pathogenesis of stress-associated skin disorders. Arch Dermatol 2001;137:53–59.
31 Kiecolt-Glaser JK, Marucha PT, Malarkey WB, Mercado AM, Glaser R: Slowing of wound healing by psychological stress. Lancet 1995;346:1194–1196.
32 Gupta MA, Gupta AK: Psychiatric and psychological co-morbidity in patients with dermatologic disorders: epidemiology and management. Am J Clin Dermatol 2003;4:833–842.
33 Picardi A, Abeni D, Melchi CF, Puddu P, Pasquini P: Psychiatric morbidity in dermatological outpatients: an issue to be recognized. Br J Dermatol 2000;143:983–991.
34 Picardi A, Pasquini P, Abeni D, Fassone G, Mazzotti E, Fava GA: Psychosomatic assessment of skin diseases in clinical practice. Psychother Psychosom 2005;74:315–322.
35 Hughes JE, Barraclough BM, Hamblin LG, White JE: Psychiatric symptoms in dermatology patients. Br J Psychiatry 1983;143:51–54.
36 Wolkenstein P, Zeller J, Revuz J, Ecosse E, Leplege A: Visibility of neurofibromatosis 1 and psychiatric morbidity. Arch Dermatol 2003;139:103–104.
37 Picardi A, Abeni D, Renzi C, Braga M, Puddu P, Pasquini P: Increased psychiatric morbidity in female outpatients with skin lesions on visible parts of the body. Acta Derm Venereol 2001;81:410–414.
38 Wessely SC, Lewis GH: The classification of psychiatric morbidity in attenders at a dermatology clinic. Br J Psychiatry 1989;155:686–691.
39 Aktan S, Ozmen E, Sanli B: Psychiatric disorders in patients attending a dermatology outpatient clinic. Dermatology 1998;197:230–234.
40 Niemeier V, Harth W, Kupfer J, Mayer K, Linse R, Schill WB, Gieler U: Prevalence of psychosomatic disorders in dermatologic patients. Experiences in 2 dermatology clinics with a liaison therapy model. Hautarzt 2002;53:471–477.
41 Dehen L, Taieb C, Myon E, Dubertret L: Dermatosis and depressive symptoms. Ann Dermatol Venereol 2006;133:125–129.
42 Attah Johnson FY, Mostaghimi H: Co-morbidity between dermatologic diseases and psychiatric disorders in Papua New Guinea. Int J Dermatol 1995;34:244–248.
43 Cohen AD, Ofek-Shlomai A, Vardy DA, Weiner Z, Shvartzman P: Depression in dermatological patients identified by the Mini International Neuropsychiatric Interview Questionnaire. J Am Acad Dermatol 2006;54:94–99.
44 Colón EA, Popkin MK, Callies AL, Dessert NJ, Hordinsky MK: Lifetime prevalence of psychiatric disorders in patients with alopecia areata. Compr Psychiatry 1991;32:245–251.
45 Kent G, Al'Abadie M: Psychologic effects of vitiligo: a critical incident analysis. J Am Acad Dermatol 1996;35:895–898.
46 Koo JY, Shellow WV, Hallman CP, Edwards JE: Alopecia areata and increased prevalence of psychiatric disorders. Int J Dermatol 1994;33:849–850.
47 Sheehan-Dare RA, Henderson MJ, Cotterill JA: Anxiety and depression in patients with chronic urticaria and generalized pruritus. Br J Dermatol 1990;123:769–774.
48 Gupta MA, Gupta AK: Depression and suicidal ideation in dermatology patients with acne, alopecia areata, atopic dermatitis and psoriasis. Br J Dermatol 1998;139:846–850.
49 Mattoo SK, Handa S, Kaur I, Gupta N, Malhotra R: Psychiatric morbidity in vitiligo and psoriasis: a comparative study from India. J Dermatol 2001;28:424–432.
50 Aktan S, Ozmen E, Sanli B: Anxiety, depression, and nature of acne vulgaris in adolescents. Int J Dermatol 2000;39:354–357.
51 Schneider G, Driesch G, Heuft G, Evers S, Luger TA, Stander S: Psychosomatic cofactors and psychiatric comorbidity in patients with chronic itch. Clin Exp Dermatol 2006;31:762–767.

52 Esposito M, Saraceno R, Giunta A, Maccarone M, Chimenti S: An Italian study on psoriasis and depression. Dermatology 2006;212:123–127.
53 Picardi A, Mazzotti E, Pasquini P: Prevalence and correlates of suicidal ideation among patients with skin disease. J Am Acad Dermatol Venereol 2006;54:420–426.
54 Zachariae R, Zachariae C, Ibsen HHW, Mortensen JT, Wulf HC: Psychological symptoms and quality of life of dermatology outpatients and hospitalized dermatology patients. Acta Derm Venereol 2004;84:205–212.
55 Khan MZ, Naeem A, Mufti KA: Prevalence of mental health problems in acne patients. J Ayub Med Coll Abbottabad 2001;13:7–8.
56 Gieler U: Psychosomatische Aspekte der Akne. Hautarzt 1988;39(suppl VIII):117–118.
57 Cotterill JA, Cunliffe WJ: Suicide in dermatological patients. Br J Dermatol 1997;137:246–250.
58 Humphreys F, Humphreys MS: Psychiatric morbidity and skin disease: what dermatologists think they see. Br J Dermatol 1998;139:679–681.
59 Staubach P, Eckhardt-Henn A, Dechene M, Vonend A, Metz M, Magerl M, Breuer P, Maurer M: Quality of life in patients with chronic urticaria is differentially impaired and determined by psychiatric comorbidity. Br J Dermatol 2006;154:294–298.
60 Sampogna F, Picardi A, Chren MM, Melchi CF, Pasquini P, Masini C, Abeni D: Association between poorer quality of life and psychiatric morbidity in patients with different dermatological conditions. Psychosom Med 2004;66:620–624.
61 Gupta MA, Gupta AK, Schork NJ, Ellis CN: Depression modulates pruritus perception: a study of pruritus in psoriasis, atopic dermatitis, and chronic idiopathic urticaria. Psychosom Med 1994;56:36–40.
62 Yosipovitch G, Ansari N, Goon A, Chan YH, Goh CL: Clinical characteristics of pruritus in chronic idiopathic urticaria. Br J Dermatol 2002;147:32–36.
63 Reich A, Szepietowski JC, Wisnicka B, Pacan P: Does stress influence itching in psoriatic patients? Dermatol Psychosom 2003;4:151–155.
64 Gupta MA, Gupta AK: Stressful major life events are associated with a higher frequency of cutaneous sensory symptoms: an empirical study of non-clinical subjects. J Eur Acad Dermatol Venereol 2004;18:560–565.
65 Renzi C, Picardi A, Abeni D, Agostini E, Baliva G, Pasquini P, Puddu P, Braga M: Association of dissatisfaction with care and psychiatric morbidity with poor treatment compliance. Arch Dermatol 2002;138:337–342.
66 Picardi A, Porcelli P, Pasquini P, Fassone G, Mazzotti E, Lega I, Ramieri L, Sagoni E, Abeni D, Tiago A, Fava GA: Integration of multiple criteria for psychosomatic assessment of dermatological patients. Psychosomatics 2006;47:122–128.
67 Wu SF, Kinder BN, Trunnell TN, Fulton JE: Role of anxiety and anger in acne patients: a relationship with the severity of the disorder. J Am Acad Dermatol 1988;18:325–333.
68 Rapp DA, Brenes GA, Feldman SR, Fleischer AB, Graham GF, Dailey M, Rapp SR: Anger and acne: implications for quality of life, patient satisfaction and clinical care. Br J Dermatol 2004;151:183–189.
69 Fried RG, Friedman S, Paradis C, Hatch M, Lynfield Y, Duncanson C, Shalita A: Trivial or terrible? The psychosocial impact of psoriasis. Int J Dermatol 1995;34:101–105.
70 Ginsburg IH, Prystowsky JH, Kornfeld DS, Wolland H: Role of emotional factors in adults with atopic dermatitis. Int J Dermatol 1993;32:656–660.
71 Conroy RM, Smyth O, Siriwardena R, Fernandes P: Health anxiety and characteristics of self-initiated general practitioner consultations. J Psychosom Res 1999;46:45–50.
72 Kellner R: Somatization and Hypochondriasis. New York, Praeger, 1986.
73 Picardi A, Porcelli P, Mazzotti E, Fassone G, Lega I, Ramieri L, Sagoni E, Pasquini P: Alexithymia and global psychosocial functioning: a study on patients with skin disease. J Psychosom Res 2007;62:223–229.
74 Krejci-Manwaring J, Kerchner K, Feldman SR, Rapp DA, Rapp SR: Social sensitivity and acne: the role of personality in negative social consequences and quality of life. Int J Psychiatry Med 2006;36:121–130.
75 Fava GA, Perini GI, Santonastaso P, Veller Fornasa C: Life events and psychological distress in dermatologic disorders: psoriasis, chronic urticaria and fungal infections. Br J Med Psychol 1980;53:277–282.

76 Lyketsos GC, Stratigos GC, Tawil G, Psaras M, Lyketsos CG: Hostile personality characteristics, dysthymic states and neurotic symptoms in urticaria, psoriasis and alopecia. Psychother Psychosom 1985;44:122–131.
77 Perini GI, Veller Fornasa C, Cipriani R, Bettin A, Zecchino F, Peserico A: Life events and alopecia areata. Psychother Psychosom 1984;41:48–52.
78 Papadopoulos L, Bor R, Legg C, Hawk JL: Impact of life events on the onset of vitiligo in adults: preliminary evidence for a psychological dimension in aetiology. Clin Exp Dermatol 1998;23: 243–248.
79 Naldi L, Chatenoud L, Linder D, Belloni Fortina A, Peserico A, Virgili AR, Bruni PL, Ingordo V, Lo Scocco G, Solaroli C, Schena D, Barba A, Di Landro A, Pezzarossa E, Arcangeli F, Gianni C, Betti R, Carli P, Farris A, Barabino GF, La Vecchia C: Cigarette smoking, body mass index, and stressful life events as risk factors for psoriasis: results from an Italian case-control study. J Invest Dermatol 2005;125:61–67.
80 Gaston L, Lassonde M, Bernier-Buzzanga J, Hodgins S, Crombez JC: Psoriasis and stress: a prospective study. J Am Acad Dermatol 1987;17:82–86.
81 King RM, Wilson GV: Use of a diary technique to investigate psychosomatic relations in atopic dermatitis. J Psychosom Res 1991;35:697–706.
82 Chiu A, Chon SY, Kimball AB: The response of skin disease to stress: changes in the severity of acne vulgaris as affected by examination stress. Arch Dermatol 2003;139:897–900.
83 Picardi A, Abeni D, Renzi C, Braga M, Melchi CF, Pasquini P: Treatment outcome and incidence of psychiatric disorders in dermatological outpatients. J Eur Acad Dermatol Venereol 2003;17: 155–159.
84 Richards HL, Fortune DG, Griffiths CE, Main CJ: The contribution of perceptions of stigmatisation to disability in patients with psoriasis. J Psychosom Res 2001;50:11–15.
85 Wittkowski A, Richards HL, Griffiths CE, Main CJ: The impact of psychological and clinical factors on quality of life in individuals with atopic dermatitis. J Psychosom Res 2004;57: 195–200.
86 Schmid-Ott G, Kunsebeck HW, Jager B, Sittig U, Hofste N, Ott R, Malewski P, Lamprecht F: Significance of the stigmatization experience of psoriasis patients: A 1-year follow-up of the illness and its psychosocial consequences in men and women. Acta Derm Venereol 2005;85:27–32.
87 Ginsburg IH, Link BG: Feelings of stigmatization in patients with psoriasis. J Am Acad Dermatol 1989;20:53–63.
88 Gupta MA, Gupta AK: The Psoriasis Life Stress Inventory: A preliminary index of psoriasis-related stress. Acta Derm Venereol 1995;75:240–243.
89 Fortune DG, Richards HL, Griffiths CE, Main CJ: Psychological stress, distress and disability in patients with psoriasis: consensus and variation in the contribution of illness perceptions, coping and alexithymia. Br J Clin Psychol 2002;41:157–174.
90 Van Moffaert M: Psychodermatology: an overview. Psychother Psychosom 1992;58:125–136.
91 Gupta MA, Gupta AK, Ellis CN, Koblenzer CS: Psychiatric evaluation of the dermatology patient. Dermatol Clin 2005;23:591–599.
92 Koblenzer CS: Dermatitis artefacta. Clinical features and approaches to treatment. Am J Clin Dermatol 2000;1:47–55.
93 Hautmann G, Hercogova J, Lotti T: Trichotillomania. J Am Acad Dermatol 2002;46:807–821.
94 Sampogna F, Picardi A, Melchi CF, Pasquini P, Abeni D: The impact of skin diseases on patients: comparing dermatologists' opinions with research data collected on their patients. Br J Dermatol 2003;148:989–995.
95 Thompson A: Coping with chronic skin conditions: factors important in explaining individual variation in adjustment; in Walker C, Papadopoulos L (eds): Psychodermatology. Cambridge, Cambridge University Press, 2005.
96 Picardi A, Amerio P, Baliva G, Barbieri C, Teofoli P, Bolli S, Salvatori V, Mazzotti E, Pasquini P, Abeni D: Recognition of depressive and anxiety disorders in dermatological outpatients. Acta Derm Venereol 2004;84:213–217.
97 Richards HL, Fortune DG, Weidmann A, Sweeney SK, Griffiths CE: Detection of psychological distress in patients with psoriasis: low consensus between dermatologist and patient. Br J Dermatol 2004;151:1227–1233.

98 Rutz W, Walinder J, Eberhard G, Holmberg G, von Knorring AL, von Knorring L, Wistedt B, Aberg-Wistedt A: An educational program on depressive disorders for general practitioners on Gotland: background and evaluation. Acta Psychiatr Scand 1989;79:19–26.
99 Gould WM: Teaching psychocutaneous medicine: time for a reappraisal. Arch Dermatol 2004;140:282–284.
100 Picardi A, Abeni D, Pasquini P: Assessing psychological distress in patients with skin diseases: reliability, validity and factor structure of the GHQ-12. J Eur Acad Dermatol Venereol 2001;15: 410–417.
101 Picardi A, Abeni D, Mazzotti E, Fassone G, Lega I, Ramieri L, Sagoni E, Tiago A, Pasquini P: Screening for psychiatric disorders in patients with skin diseases: a performance study of the 12-item General Health Questionnaire. J Psychosom Res 2004;57:219–223.
102 Picardi A, Adler DA, Abeni D, Chang H, Pasquini P, Rogers WH, Bungay KM: Screening for depressive disorders in patients with skin diseases: a comparison of three screeners. Acta Derm Venereol 2005;85:414–419.
103 Worrall G, Angel J, Chaulk P, Clarke C, Robbins M: Effectiveness of an educational strategy to improve family physicians' detection and management of depression: a randomized controlled trial. Can Med Assoc J 1999;61:37–40.
104 Gilbody SM, Whitty PM, Grimshaw JM, Thomas RE: Improving the detection and management of depression in primary care. Qual Saf Health Care 2003;12:149–155.
105 Palmer SC, Coyne JC: Screening for depression in medical care: pitfalls, alternatives, and revised priorities. J Psychosom Res 2003;54:279–287.
106 Gould WM, Gragg TM: A dermatology-psychiatry liaison clinic. J Am Acad Dermatol 1983;9:73–77.
107 de Korte J, Van Onselen J, Kownacki S, Sprangers MA, Bos JD: Quality of care in patients with psoriasis: an initial clinical study of an international disease management programme. J Eur Acad Dermatol Venereol 2005;19:35–41.
108 Millard L: Dermatological practice and psychiatry. Br J Dermatol 2000;143:920–921.
109 Fortune DG, Richards HL, Kirby B, McElhone K, Markham T, Rogers S, Main CJ, Griffiths CE: Psychological distress impairs clearance of psoriasis in patients treated with photochemotherapy. Arch Dermatol 2003;139:752–756.
110 Fortune DG, Richards HL, Kirby B, Bowcock S, Main CJ, Griffiths CE: A cognitive-behavioural symptom management programme as an adjunct in psoriasis therapy. Br J Dermatol 2002;146: 458–465.
111 Kabat-Zinn J, Wheeler E, Light T, Skillings A, Scharf MJ, Cropley TG, Hosmer D, Bernhard JD: Influence of a mindfulness meditation-based stress reduction intervention on rates of skin clearing in patients with moderate to severe psoriasis undergoing phototherapy (UVB) and photochemotherapy (PUVA). Psychosom Med 1998;60:625–632.
112 Fortune DG, Richards HL, Kirby B, McElhone K, Main CJ, Griffiths CEM: Successful treatment of psoriasis improves psoriasis-specific but not more general aspects of patients' well-being. Br J Dermatol 2004;151:1219–1226.
113 Woodruff PW, Higgins EM, du Vivier AW, Wessely S: Psychiatric illness in patients referred to a dermatology-psychiatry clinic. Gen Hosp Psychiatry 1997;19:29–35.
114 Folks DG, Kinney FC: The role of psychological-factors in dermatological conditions. Psychosomatics 1992;33:45–54.

Dr. Angelo Picardi
Italian National Institute of Health, Centre of Epidemiology
Surveillance and Health Promotion
Viale Regina Elena, 299
IT–00161 Rome (Italy)
Tel. +39 06 4990 4200, Fax +39 06 4990 4182, E-Mail angelo.picardi@iss.it

Porcelli P, Sonino N (eds): Psychological Factors Affecting Medical Conditions. A New Classification for DSM-V. Adv Psychosom Med. Basel, Karger, 2007, vol 28, pp 127–140

Psychological Factors Affecting Medical Conditions in Consultation-Liaison Psychiatry

Antonello Bellomo[a], *Mario Altamura*[a], *Antonio Ventriglio*[a], *Angelo Rella*[b], *Roberto Quartesan*[b], *Sandro Elisei*[b]

[a]Section of Psychiatry and Clinical Psychology, Department of Medical Sciences, University of Foggia, Foggia, [b]Section of Psychiatry, Clinical Psychology and Psychiatric Rehabilitation, Department of Clinical and Experimental Medicine, University of Perugia, Perugia, Italy

Abstract

Consultation-liaison (C-L) psychiatry has an important role in the identification and management of psychological problems in patients with medical disorders in general hospitals. The diagnostic tools C-L psychiatrists are usually provided with may reveal to be limited because of particular psychosomatic syndromes and subthreshold psychopathology that are undetected by psychiatric diagnostic criteria. The Diagnostic Criteria for Psychosomatic Research (DCPR) were developed with the aim of providing clinicians with operational criteria for psychosomatic syndromes to overcome the limitations shown by the most often diagnosed disorders in medical settings as adjustment, somatoform, mood, and anxiety disorders. In a group of 66 consecutive C-L psychiatry inpatients, a consistent prevalence of 71% DCPR syndromes was found, particularly secondary functional somatic symptoms, persistent somatization, health anxiety, and demoralization. Their overlap rates with DSM-IV diagnoses showed that the DCPR syndromes were able to identify psychological dimensions (as somatic symptom clustering, anxiety triggered by the current health status, and a feeling state of hopelessness) that do not meet or are not detected by DSM-IV. Furthermore, the DCPR syndromes identified patients with clinically significant functional impairment. These results replicate previous findings in C-L psychiatry using the DCPR categories and pave the way for further research to clarify their mediating role in the course and the outcome variance of medical and psychological problems of hospital inpatients referred for psychiatric consultation.

The consultation-liaison (C-L) psychiatrist is called upon to evaluate and treat a wide variety of psychiatric disorders in patients with general medical conditions. However, the role of the C-L psychiatrist in clinical practice is not characterized merely by adding a piece of information (the 'mind side' of a clinical problem) to other pieces on the 'biology side', as for example it happens with a gastroenterologist asking for a consultation from a cardiologist. Psychological, social, and cultural factors are involved in various degrees in the onset, course, and outcome of pathophysiological processes [1]. Therefore the C-L psychiatrist is often faced with complex interacting determinants of the overall health status of the patient and might find the available diagnostic armamentarium as poorly adequate for the clinical reality [2].

Psychiatric Diagnoses in Medical Setting

The psychiatric taxonomy over the years has been insufficiently attentive to the way in which psychiatric diagnosis may be affected by the co-occurrence of physical illness and, in turn, physical illness may be affected by psychological factors. Somatic symptoms may overlay psychiatric symptoms to the extent that psychiatric algorithms do not apply. For instance, insomnia, lack of energy, anorexia and diminished sexual drive are symptoms common to both major depression and several medical illnesses, and it is not an easy task for a clinician to know the origin of symptoms. On the other hand, psychological mechanisms such as an obsessive cognitive pattern may be hidden by functional intestinal symptoms that in turn overlap with typical symptoms of an organic disease like ulcerative colitis [3]. Patients with several specific medical illnesses may have high rates of psychiatric comorbidity and present challenges for psychiatrists. For example, severe psychopathology may affect patients with infective disease such as acquired immune deficiency syndrome and chronic hepatitis C, including delirium, depression, and symptoms caused by opportunistic infections and antiviral drugs [4, 5]. Furthermore, more complex psychological characteristics have been recently recognized in specific medical conditions, such as atypical presentation of delirium [6], psychiatric features of several paraneoplastic syndromes [7, 8], complex presentation of depression in cancer patients [9, 10], posttraumatic states following intensive care treatment and human immunodeficiency virus infection [11]. Driven by frustration and belief system, when confronted with diagnostic ambiguity, the psychiatrist may be inclined to make unjustifiable psychiatric diagnoses such as malingering, hypochondriasis, depression, anxiety, and so on.

A further limitation of psychosocial diagnoses in the medical setting comes from the fact that many of the issues are not necessarily traditional psychiatric diagnoses, as poor adherence to treatment, bereavement or adaptation to severe illnesses. For instance, the adjustment disorders category is a diagnostic

Table 1. Rates of psychiatric diagnoses (%) made in psychiatric consultation in inpatients [adapted from 60]

Study	Country	Mood disorders	Adjustment disorders	Anxiety disorders
Karasu et al. [41]	US	21.2	3.3	4.0
Lipowski and Wolston [42]	US	50.2	n.s.	6.8
Craig [43]	US	28.6	n.s.	n.s.
Perez and Silverman [44]	Canada	36.4	15.6	0
Loewenstein and Sharfstein [45]	US	27.2	16.5	6.8
McKegney et al. [46]	US	10.0	33.0	3.0
Hengeveld et al. [47]	Netherlands	18.8	8.3	8.4
Malhotra and Malhotra [48]	India	31.3	n.s.	n.s.
Hales et al. [49]	US	14.4	18.7	1.3
Kuhn et al. [50]	US	26.0	9.0	n.s.
Schofield et al. [51]	Ireland	44.0	n.s.	n.s.
Sobel et al. [52]	Israel	15.9	3.9	6.6
Wallen et al. [53]	US	51.3	n.s.	n.s.
Clark and Smith [54]	Australia	55.0	19.0	3.0
Ramchandani et al. [55]	US	10.0	14.0	n.s.
Ormont et al. [56]	US	13.9	9.9	2.0
DeJonge et al. [57]	Europe	18.5	n.s.	18.5
Grant et al. [58]	US	56.7	n.s.	16.0
Diefenbacher and Strani [59]	US	29.8	n.s.	n.s.
Bourgeois et al. [60]	US	35.4	11.7	7.0

n.s. = Not specified.

group with questionable reliability, validity, and clinical utility [12], even though it is one of the most commonly used diagnoses in the medical setting [13]. A recent review showed that the rates of referred cases in which a psychiatric diagnosis was made ranged from 50 to 99% in seven medical specialty clinics [14]. The somatoform disorders category is another diagnostic group of questionable validity and utility. Though they should be expected to be highly prevalent in medical patients because of the high rate of functional and medically unexplained symptoms, somatoform disorders are very rarely diagnosed in medical settings, including C-L psychiatry [15] and have been widely criticized and suggested to be abolished in the DSM-V [16, 17]. Table 1 shows the prevalence rates of some common psychiatric diagnoses in general hospital medical departments, ranging from 10 to 50% for mood disorders, 3 to 19% for adjustment disorders, and 0 to 18% for anxiety disorders, according to the various medical settings, inclusion criteria, and classification systems.

It should also be underscored what is hidden in the figures shown in table 1, namely the high rate (up to 50%) of inpatients for whom a psychiatric consultation is requested but no DSM-based diagnosis was made. In fact, psychiatric diagnoses in medical settings, including hospital wards, are biased by mind-body dualism as it is evidenced in two core concepts that are dominant in the DSM-IV [18]. First, the diagnosis of somatization is often placed when somatic symptoms are likely to mimic 'real' symptoms of medical disease while not showing any evidence of it. The critical concept in this view is the distance considered as clinically excessive between the physical problem (inexistent or not being a plausible cause for actual symptoms) and the patient's perception, thoughts, and behavior. Second, the somatic symptoms should not be secondary to other psychiatric disorders. This view pertains to the concept of hierarchical organization, according to which, the somatoform symptoms are placed at the same level as other axis I syndromes. A viable alternative could consider association instead of distance, and coexistence instead of hierarchy, namely, the psychological correlates of somatic symptom reporting, regardless of the presence of other psychiatric syndromes or the questionable distinction of functional illness versus physical disease.

Assessment of Psychosocial Factors with the Diagnostic Criteria for Psychosomatic Research in Consultation-Liaison Psychiatry

Because of the shortcomings highlighted in the use of DSM-IV categories in medical setting, a more comprehensive theoretical framework and sensitive diagnostic tools are needed for the assessment of psychosocial issues in medical inpatients and C-L psychiatry. The most popular framework used to encompass all the multiple factors interacting to shape the course of medical disorders is the biopsychosocial model [19] which recognizes that psychosocial conditions may alter physiological functioning, exacerbate symptoms of medical disorders, contribute to persistence of physical symptoms, and modify the individual experience of medical illness. In turn, medical disorders may have psychosocial consequences on one's general well-being, daily functioning, and health-related quality of life. Among the guidelines for C-L psychiatrists of the Academy of Psychosomatic Medicine [20], the assessment of patients' behavior and personality styles is highly recommended. The C-L consultant is indeed suggested to assess how well the patient is coping and whether he or she is able to endure the course of the illness. Furthermore, the consultant is suggested to integrate information from several domains (e.g. developmental, social, and occupational history) to form a dynamic life narrative leading up to the current illness. However, the problem with such an overarching model is that it is very general and therefore lacks operational concepts applicable to the practical tasks of medicine [21].

The DSM-IV rubric of Psychological Factors Affecting Medical Conditions is not a viable specification of the biopsychosocial model because it lacks diagnostic validity, clinical utility and theoretical adequacy. The Diagnostic Criteria for Psychosomatic Research (DCPR) [22] provide instead a very useful framework for investigating psychological distress, psychosocial determinants, and subclinical psychopathology of patients with medical conditions. The DCPR syndromes have been used in C-L psychiatry in a study investigating their prevalence in 100 inpatients from a general hospital [23]. Only 13% of patients did not receive a DCPR diagnosis, while 25% of them failed to meet any criteria for psychiatric diagnosis made with the ICD-10 classification system. In particular, demoralization, alexithymia, and illness denial were the most prevalent DCPR diagnoses with rates of 39, 30, and 29%, respectively.

The present chapter reports preliminary data on the use of DCPR categories in medical inpatients who were referred for psychiatric consultation from two Italian general hospitals. The aim of this exploratory study was twofold. First, we aimed to replicate the findings of Galeazzi et al. [23] by using the DSM-IV classification system. Second, we aimed to evaluate whether the presence of psychological correlates of medical illness or subthreshold psychopathology in medical inpatients may result in impaired psychosocial functioning.

The sample consisted of 66 inpatients (26 men and 40 women, mean age 44.4 ± 13.3, mean education years 9.4 ± 3.2) who were consecutively recruited from among those referred for psychiatric consultation to the C-L psychiatry service of two Italian university general hospitals (Perugia and Foggia). Patients were excluded if they were aged <18 and >64 years, had cognitive impairment, refused to cooperate, and had psychotic, delusional, and significant physical pain symptoms. All patients agreed to participate and gave their informed consent. Sociodemographic data, medical information, and psychopathology (self-reported psychiatric diagnosis received recently or in the past 10 years, psychiatric or psychological treatments received in the past 10 years) were collected. Each patient received a psychiatric diagnosis through the Italian version of the Structured Clinical Interview for DSM-IV [24, 25] and a psychosomatic diagnosis through the Italian translation of the Interview for the DCPR [26]. Because of lower reliability information, the DCPR category of alexithymia was excluded from the analysis. Psychosocial functioning was assessed with the Italian version of the Medical Outcomes Study 36-Item Short Form (SF-36) [27, 28]. The SF-36 consists of eight scales that correspond to the main domains of functional status and well-being, including health limitations of physical activities (Physical functioning), physical health limitations on work and other daily responsibilities (Role functioning – physical), intensity of bodily pain or discomfort (Bodily pain), subjective perception of health status (General health), physical energy and fatigue (Vitality), impact of health or emotional problems on social activities (Social functioning), mental health limitations on work and other daily responsibilities (Role functioning – emotional), and subjective psychological well-being (Mental health). Two composite scores are also obtained for evaluating the Physical Component Scale and the Mental Component Scale of the quality of life. The characteristics of the sample are shown in table 2.

Most patients were diagnosed with at least one DSM-IV category (86%). However, consistently with other studies [29], only one third of them (36%) reported current or lifetime psychiatric problems, suggesting that psychopathology might have been underestimated by the treating physician, psychological symptoms might have overlapped with somatic illness, patients might underreport their psychological problems to their physicians, or they suffered from subclinical symptoms. Forty out of 57 (70.2%) patients diagnosed with DSM-IV disorders reported lifetime and current psychopathology. The most prevalent DSM-IV diagnostic groups were adjustment (26%), anxiety (23%), and mood disorders (18%). Only 10 patients (15%) were diagnosed with one of the somatoform disorders. The figures are quite consistent with those reported by Galeazzi et al. [23] who found 54% patients with ICD-10 F4 category (anxiety, dissociative, stress-related, somatoform, and other nonpsychotic mental disorders) that comprises syndromes classified as adjustment, anxiety, and somatoform disorders in the DSM-IV, and 12% with ICD-10 F3 category (affective disorders).

A total of 71% of patients received at least one and 35 (53%) more than one DCPR diagnosis. The most prevalent DCPR diagnoses were functional somatic symptoms secondary to psychopathology (36%), health anxiety (30%), persistent somatization (23%), and demoralization (23%). Compared to our results, Galeazzi et al. [23] found higher prevalence of at least one DCPR (87%) but lower prevalence of single DCPR diagnoses, with demoralization (18%), alexithymia (13%), and illness denial (13%) as the most prevalent DCPR categories. Differences between the results of the two studies might be due to the sample characteristics (differences in sociocultural living contexts and younger age in our patients) and the use of different psychiatric classification systems (DSM-IV and ICD-10).

Tables 3 and 4 show the overlapping rates between DSM-IV and DCPR diagnoses in our sample.

Large proportions of patients diagnosed with mood and anxiety disorders had also functional somatic symptoms secondary to the psychopathological conditions (50 and 73%, respectively), much more than the parent DCPR categories of demoralization for mood disorders (42%) and health anxiety for

Table 2. Psychiatric and psychosomatic characteristics of C-L psychiatric patients

	n	%
Medical settings		
Gastroenterology	19	28.7
Internal medicine	11	16.6
Dermatology	9	13.6
Work medicine	8	12.1
Infective disease	6	9.1
Neurology	6	9.1
Others	7	10.6
Psychopathology		
Adjustment disorders	17	25.7
Anxiety disorders	15	22.7
Mood disorders	12	18.2
Somatoform disorders	10	15.1
Others	3	4.5
Any DSM-IV disorders	57	86.4
Self-reported psychiatric disorders	24	36.3
DCPR diagnoses		
Functional somatic symptoms secondary to a psychiatric disorder	24	36.4
Health anxiety	20	30.3
Persistent somatization	15	22.7
Demoralization	15	22.7
Disease phobia	8	12.1
Illness denial	8	12.1
Type A behavior	7	10.6
Irritable mood	7	10.6
Conversion symptoms	4	6.1
Anniversary reaction	4	6.1
Thanatophobia	1	1.5
Any DCPR syndrome	47	71.2
>1 DCPR diagnosis	35	53.0

anxiety disorders (40%). Both mood and anxiety disorders overlapped also with persistent somatization (33%) (table 3). Moreover, patients with the most prevalent DCPR syndromes met the criteria for DSM-IV disorders (table 4). Of interest, large proportions of patients with DCPR syndromes were not classified by DSM-IV and no overlap was found between persistent somatization and

Table 3. Overlapping rates of DCPR categories in patients meeting criteria for DSM-IV diagnoses

	FSS	Health anxiety	Persistent somatization	Demoralization
Adjustment disorders (n = 17)	17.6	23.5	0	35.3
Anxiety disorders (n = 15)	73.3	40.0	33.3	13.3
Mood disorders (n = 12)	50.0	16.7	33.3	41.7

FSS = Functional somatic symptoms secondary to a psychiatric disorder.

Table 4. Overlapping rates of DSM-IV diagnoses in patients meeting criteria for DCPR categories

	FSS (n = 24)	Health anxiety (n = 20)	Persistent somatization (n = 15)	Demoralization (n = 15)
Adjustment disorders	12.5	20.0	0	40.0
Anxiety disorders	45.8	30.0	33.3	13.3
Mood disorders	25.0	10.0	26.7	33.3

adjustment disorders. These findings are substantially consistent with those obtained by Galeazzi et al. [23] and two studies on demoralization [30] and adjustment disorders [12].

The role of DCPR syndromes in psychosocial functioning was explored by analyzing the difference in SF-36 scale scores between patients with (n = 47) and without (n = 19) DCPR diagnoses (fig. 1).

Overall, except for Vitality and General health (assessing physical health and energy), all SF-36 scales were lower in patients with DCPR compared to those without DCPR, suggesting poorer psychosocial functioning. Statistically significant differences were found for Social functioning (interference of physical and emotional problems with normal social activities; $t = 2.34$, $p < 0.05$; effect size = 0.28), Role functioning – emotional (problems with work or other daily activities as a result of emotional problems; $t = 2.31$, $p < 0.05$; effect

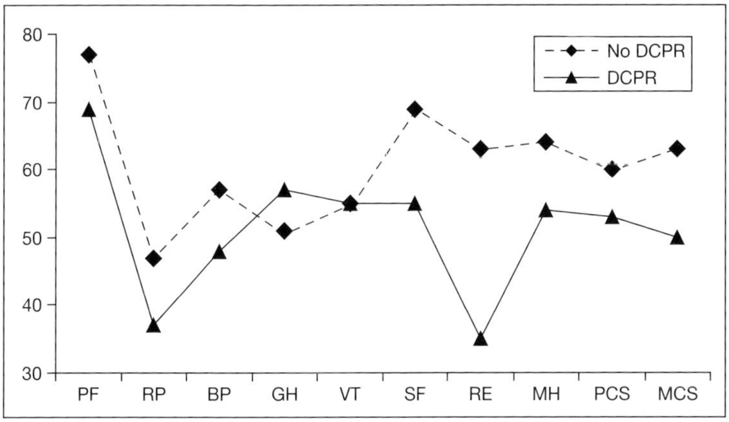

Fig. 1. SF-36 scores of patients with (n = 47) and without (n = 19) DCPR diagnoses.

size = 0.28), Mental health (feelings of nervousness and depression; t = 2.11, $p < 0.05$; effect size = 0.26), and Mental Component Scale (psychological distress and social disability due to emotional problems; t = 2.42, $p < 0.05$; effect size = 0.29) that were worse in patients with DCPR. Since all patients were hospitalized because of their physical illness and the physical health-related scales of the SF-36, including the composite Physical Component Scale score, were similar in the two groups, these results suggest that the presence of DCPR-related problems greatly affected mental adjustment to disease and adaptive coping attitude. Our findings are consistent with those obtained in studies using DCPR and measures of psychosocial functioning in patients with endocrine disease [31] and in subjects from a community sample [32].

Clinical Implications of the Use of the DCPR in Consultation-Liaison Psychiatry

A recent meta-review showed that many areas of C-L psychiatry practice are not based on high-quality evidence [33]. One of the most important flaws is represented by the extrapolation of methods from other areas of psychiatry where there is high-quality evidence. For instance, a review of antidepressant treatment in medical patients combined the results of clinical trials of treatments for depression in a wide range of physical illnesses [34]. Even though the efficacy of antidepressants is well demonstrated in homogeneous samples of psychiatric patients, clinical heterogeneity may hamper the extrapolation of the same treatment to somatic patients, who may also experience very negative effects from antidepressant medications [35].

The need for a more comprehensive taxonomy in psychiatry, particularly when applied to the medical setting, was evidenced by McHugh and Slavney [36] who encouraged psychiatrists to pay attention to psychological mechanisms beyond the mere appearance of symptoms, particularly to the dimensions of etiology (focusing on the clinical syndrome rather than just observable phenomena), cognition and affects (focusing on coping mechanisms with life demands), behavior (focusing on the ability to control over drives and preoccupations), and narrative (focusing on the individual life history, experiences, and perceptions). McHuge and Slavney's call for a true diagnostic approach in psychiatry is in line with the need for an integrative multidisciplinary framework in modern psychosomatic medicine [37, 38]. The DCPR classification is a reliable tool for investigating those aspects that cannot be identified by the DSM-IV criteria because either they are not present at all in that system (as type A behavior) or are subsyndromal and do not meet the DSM-IV stringent criteria (as health anxiety and persistent somatization) or are underestimated by the hierarchical principle of the DSM-IV approach (as functional somatic symptoms secondary to a psychiatric disorder). Our results and those of Galeazzi et al. [23] clearly show that the DCPR can be used in C-L psychiatry setting and reliably identify psychological problems in medical patients that are not included in the criteria for the most used DSM-IV categories in medical settings as somatoform, adjustment, mood, and anxiety disorders.

Among the 4 most prevalent DCPR psychosomatic syndromes found in the present study, secondary functional somatic symptoms and persistent somatization can be conceived as substitutes of somatization and undifferentiated somatoform disorders. The category of secondary functional somatic symptoms is used when these physical ailments are subsequent to psychiatric symptoms and therefore bypass the hierarchical principle of DSM-IV and the category of persistent somatization is used when the patient suffers from multiple somatic symptoms in the previous 6 months or exaggerated side effects from medical therapy. They are issued from Kellner's [39] concept of the somatizing patient as someone in whom psychosomatic symptoms have clustered. In our sample, the prevalence of these two DCPR syndromes was about twice that of all the diagnostic categories of the somatoform disorder rubric. Another frequent DCPR category in our sample was demoralization, which is very common in the medically ill [31]. Demoralization is different from clinical depression, adjustment disorder with depressed mood and subthreshold depression, as confirmed by our finding that only 40% of patients with adjustment disorders, 33% with mood disorders, and 13% with anxiety disorders also had DCRP demoralization. Finally, the DCPR criteria of health anxiety require that the subject is highly concerned with health worries and fears for having a serious disease, as in the DSM-IV hypochondriasis, but this feeling state is of short duration and is easily reduced by appropriate medical explanations on the nature of the physical symptoms. Although it can be viewed as a form of somatic stress or generalized anxiety or depressive focus on the subject's physical concerns, we found that 60% of patients with health anxiety did not meet the criteria for any anxiety disorders, 83% for any mood disorders, and 77% for adjustment disorders. The identification of these psychological syndromes in medical inpatients referred to C-L psychiatry may have important implications for clinical management because they have been found to be significant predictors of treatment outcome in patients with functional gastrointestinal disorders [40].

In conclusion, findings available so far indicate that the DCPR can provide the C-L psychiatrist with a set of diagnostic criteria that are more sensitive and comprehensive than the usual psychiatric taxonomy, more specific and operational than the popular biopsychosocial model, and able to investigate functional impairment. There is a need for further research in order to clarify the mediating role of DCPR in the course and the outcome variance of medical and psychological problems of hospital inpatients referred for psychiatric consultation.

References

1 Fava GA, Mangelli L, Ruini C: Assessment of psychological distress in the setting of medical disease. Psychother Psychosom 2001;70:171–175.
2 Strain JJ: Psychiatric diagnostic dilemmas in the medical setting. Aust N Z J Psychiatry 2005;3–9: 764–771.
3 Porcelli P, Leandro G: Bowel obsession syndrome in a patient with ulcerative colitis. Psychosomatics 2007, in press.
4 Dube B, Benton T, Cruess DG, Evans DL: Neuropsychiatric manifestations of HIV infection and AIDS. J Psychiatry Neurosci 2005;30:237–246.
5 Lim JK, Cronkite R, Goldstein MK, Cheung RC: The impact of chronic hepatitis C and comorbid psychiatric illnesses on health-related quality of life. J Clin Gastroenterol 2006;40:528–534.
6 Stagno D, Gibson C, Breibart W: The delirium subtypes: a review of prevalence, phenomenology, pathophysiology, and treatment response. Palliat Support Care 2004;2:171–179.
7 Schonfeldt-Leucona C, Freudenmann RW, Tumani H, Kassubek J, Connemann BJ: Acute psychosis with a mediastinal carcinoma metastasis. Med Sci Monit 2005;11:CS6–CS8.
8 Muehlschlegel S, Okun MS, Foote KD, Coco D, Yachnis AT, Fernandez HH: Paraneoplastic chorea with leukoencephalophathy presenting obsessive-compulsive and behavioural disorders. Mov Disord 2005;20:1523–1527.
9 Pessin H, Olden M, Jacobson C, Kosinski A: Clinical assessment of depression in terminally ill cancer patients: a practical guide. Palliat Support Care 2005;3:319–324.
10 Jacobsen JC, Vanderwerker L, Block S, Friedlander R, Maciejewski P, Prigerson H: Depression and demoralization as distinct syndromes: preliminary data from a cohort of advanced cancer patients. Indian J Palliat Care 2006;12:8–15.
11 Tedstone JE, Tarrier N: Postraumatic stress disorder following medical illness and treatment. Clin Psychol Rev 2003;23:409–448.

12 Grassi L, Mangelli L, Fava GA, Grandi S, Ottolini F, Porcelli P, Rafanelli C, Rigatelli M, Sonino N: Psychosomatic characterization of adjustment disorders in the medical setting. Some suggestions for DSM-V. J Affect Dis 2007, in press.
13 Strain JS, Smith GC, Hammer JS, McKenzie DP, Blumenfield M, Muskin P, Newstadt G, Wallack J, Wilner A, Schleifer SS: Adjustment disorder: a multisite study of its utilization and interventions in the Consultation-Liaison psychiatry setting. Gen Hosp Psychiatry 1998;20:139–149.
14 Nimnuan C, Hotopf M, Wessely S: Medically unexplained symptoms: an epidemiological study in seven specialities. J Psychosom Res 2001;51:361–367.
15 Thomassen R, van Hemert AM, Huyse FJ, van der Mast RC, Hengeveld MW: Somatoform disorders in consultation-liaison psychiatry: a comparison with other mental disorders. Gen Hosp Psychiatry 2003;25:8–13.
16 Mayou R, Kirmayer LJ, Simon G, Kroenke K, Sharpe M: Somatoform disorders: time for a new approach in DSM-V. Am J Psychiatry 2005;162:847–855.
17 Fava GA, Wise T: Psychological factors affecting either identified or feared medical conditions: a solution for somatoform disorders in DSM-V. Am J Psychiatry 2007, in press.
18 Porcelli P, Mangelli L: Somatoform disorders. New approaches to classification, conceptualization, and treatment (letter). J Psychosom Res 2005;58:211–212.
19 Engel GL: The clinical application of the biopsychosocial model. Am J Psychiatry 1980;137: 535–544.
20 Bronheim HE, Fulop G, Kunkel EJ, Muskin PR, Schindler BA, Yates WR, Shaw R, Steiner H, Stern TA, Stoudemire A: The Academy of Psychosomatic Medicine Practice Guidelines for psychiatric consultation in the general medical setting. Psychosomatics 1998;39:S8–S30.
21 Oken D: Multiaxial diagnosis and psychosomatic model of disease. Psychosom Med 2000;62: 171–175.
22 Fava GA, Freyberger HJ, Bech P, Christodoulou G, Sensky T, Theorell T, Wise TN: Diagnostic criteria for use in psychosomatic research. Psychother Psychosom 1995;63:1–8.
23 Galeazzi GM, Ferrari S, Mackinnon A, Rigatelli M: Interrater reliability, prevalence, and relation to ICD-10 diagnoses of the Diagnostic Criteria for Psychosomatic Research in Consultation-Liaison psychiatry patients. Psychosomatics 2004;45:386–393.
24 First MB, Gibbon M, Spitzer RL, Williams JBW, Benjamin LS: SCID-II – Structured Clinical Interview for DSM-IV Axis II Personality Disorders (Italian version by Mazzi F, Morosini P, De Girolamo G, Guaraldi GP). Firenze, Organizzazioni Speciali, 2003.
25 First MB, Spitzer RL, Gibbon M, Williams JBW: SCID-I – Structured Clinical Interview for DSM-IV Axis I Disorders (Italian version by Mazzi F, Morosini P, De Girolamo G, Lussetti M, Guaraldi GP). Firenze, Organizzazioni Speciali, 2000.
26 Mangelli L, Rafanelli C, Porcelli P, Fava GA: Interview for the Diagnostic Criteria of Psychosomatic Research (DCPR). Psychother Psychosom 2003;72:346 –349.
27 Ware JE: SF-36 Health Survey. Manual and Interpretation Guide. Boston, New England Medical Center, 1993.
28 Apolone G, Moscati P, Ware JE: Questionario sullo stato di salute SF-36. Manuale d'uso e guida all'interpretazione dei risultati. Milano, Guerini e Associati, 1997.
29 Rentsch D, Dumont P, Borgacci S, Carballeira YC, deTonnac N, Archinard M, Andreoli A: Prevalence and treatment of depression in a hospital department of internal medicine. Gen Hosp Psychiatry 2007;29:25–31.
30 Mangelli L, Fava GA, Grandi S, Grassi L, Ottolini F, Porcelli P, Rafanelli C, Rigatelli M, Sonino N: Assessing demoralization and depression in the setting of medical disease. J Clin Psychiatry 2005; 66:391–394.
31 Sonino N, Navarrini C, Ruini C, Ottolini F, Paoletta A, Fallo F, Boscaro M, Fava GA: Persistent psychological distress in patients treated for endocrine disease. Psychother Psychosom 2004;73: 78–83.
32 Mangelli L, Semprini F, Sirri L, Fava GA, Sonino N: Use of the Diagnostic Criteria for Psychosomatic Research (DCPR) in a community sample. Psychosomatics 2006;47:143–146.
33 Ruddy R, House A: Meta-review of high-quality systematic reviews of interventions in key areas of liaison psychiatry. Br J Psychiatry 2005;187:109–120.

34 Gill D, Hatcher S: Antidepressants for depression in medical illnesses. Cochrane Database Syst Rev 2002;4.
35 Looper KJ: Potential medical and surgical complications of serotonergic antidepressant medications. Psychosomatics 2007;48:1–9.
36 McHugh PR, Slavney PR: The Perspectives of Psychiatry, ed 2. Baltimore, John Hopkins University Press, 1998.
37 Wise TN: Consultation liaison psychiatry and psychosomatics: strange bedfellows. Psychother Psychosom 2000;69.181–183.
38 Fava GA, Sonino N: The clinical domains of psychosomatic medicine. J Clin Psychiatry 2005;66:849–858.
39 Kellner R: Psychosomatic syndromes and somatic symptoms. Washington, American Psychiatric Press, 1991.
40 Porcelli P, De Carne M, Todarello O: The prediction of treatment outcome of patients with functional gastrointestinal disorders by the Diagnostic Criteria for Psychosomatic Research (DCPR). Psychother Psychosom 2004;73:166–173.
41 Karasu TB, Plutchik R, Steinmuller RI, Conte H, Siegel B: Patterns of psychiatric consultation in a general hospital. Hosp Community Psychiatry 1977;28:291–294.
42 Lipowski ZJ, Wolston EJ: Liaison psychiatry: referral patterns and their stability over time. Am J Psychiatry 1981;138:1608–1611.
43 Craig TJ: An epidemiologic study of a psychiatric liaison service. Gen Hosp Psychiatry 1982;4: 131–137.
44 Perez EL, Silverman M: Utilization pattern of a Canadian psychiatric consultation service. Gen Hosp Psychiatry 1983;5:185–190.
45 Loewenstein RJ, Sharfstein SS: Psychiatric consultations at the NIMH. Gen Hosp Psychiatry 1983;5:83–87.
46 McKegney FP, McMahon T, King J: The use of DSM-III in a general hospital consultation-liaison service. Gen Hosp Psychiatry 1983;5:115–121.
47 Hengeveld MW, Rooymans HGM, Vecht-van den Bergh R: Psychiatric consultations in a Dutch university hospital: a report on 1814 referrals, compared with a literature review. Gen Hosp Psychiatry 1984;6:271–279.
48 Malhotra S, Malhotra A: Liaison psychiatry in an Indian general hospital. Gen Hosp Psychiatry 1984;6:266–270.
49 Hales RE, Polly S, Bridenbaugh H, Orman D: Psychiatric consultations in a military hospital: a report on 1065 cases. Gen Hosp Psychiatry 1986;8:173–182.
50 Kuhn WG, Bell RA, Frierson RL, Lippman SB: Consultative psychiatry in both private and public general hospitals. Gen Hosp Psychiatry 1986;8:236–240.
51 Schofield A, Doonan H, Daly RJ: Liaison psychiatry in an Irish hospital: a survey of a year's experience. Gen Hosp Psychiatry 1986;8:119–122.
52 Sobel SN, Munitz H, Karp L: Psychiatric consultations in two Israeli general hospitals. Gen Hosp Psychiatry 1988;10:298–304.
53 Wallen J, Pincus HA, Goldman HH, Marcus SE: Psychiatric consultations in short-term general hospitals. Arch Gen Psychiatry 1987;44:163–168.
54 Clarke DM, Smith GC: Consultation-liaison psychiatry in general medical units. Aust N Z J Psychiatry 1995;29:424–432.
55 Ramchandani D, Lamdan RM, O'Dowd MA, Boland R, Hails K, Ball S, Schindler BA: What, why, and how of consultation psychiatry: an analysis of the consultation process at five urban teaching hospitals. Psychosomatics 1997;38:349–355.
56 Ormont MA, Weisman HW, Heller SS, Najara JE, Shindledecker RD: The timing of psychiatric consultation requests: utilization, liaison, and diagnostic considerations. Psychosomatics 1997;38:38–44.
57 De Jonge P, Huyse FJ, Herzog T, Lobo A, Malt U, Opmeer BC, Kuiper B, Krabbendam A: Referral pattern of neurological patients to psychiatric consultation-liaison services in 33 European hospitals. Gen Hosp Psychiatry 2001;23:152–157.
58 Grant JE, Meller W, Urevig B: Changes in psychiatric consultations over ten years. Gen Hosp Psychiatry 2001;23:261–265.

59 Diefenbacher A, Strain JJ: Consultation-liaison psychiatry: stability and change over a 10-year-period. Gen Hosp Psychiatry 2002;24:249–256.
60 Bourgeois JA, Wegelin JA, Servis ME, Hales RE: Psychiatric diagnoses of 901 inpatients seen by Consultation-Liaison Psychiatrists at an Academic medical center in a managed Care Environment. Psychosomatics 2005;46:47–57.

Prof. Antonello Bellomo
Dipartimento di Scienze Mediche, Sezione di Psichiatria e Psicologia Clinica
Università degli Studi di Foggia
Viale L. Pinto
IT–71100 Foggia (Italy)
Tel./Fax +39 0881 732 285, E-Mail a.bellomo@unifg.it

Porcelli P, Sonino N (eds): Psychological Factors Affecting Medical Conditions. A New Classification for DSM-V. Adv Psychosom Med. Basel, Karger, 2007, vol 28, pp 141–168

Psychological Factors Affecting Eating Disorders

Secondo Fassino, Giovanni Abbate Daga, Andrea Pierò, Nadia Delsedime

Università degli Studi di Torino, Eating Disorders Centre Molinette Hospital, Torino, Italy

Abstract

Eating disorders (EDs) are representative of the relationship between psychosomatic and psychiatric disorders and have complex interactions in the body, mind, and brain. The psychosomatic issues of EDs emerge in the alterations of the body and its functioning, in personality traits, in the difficulty of recognizing and coping with emotions, and in the management of anger and impulsiveness. The Diagnostic Criteria for Psychosomatic Research used by the authors of this chapter (alexithymia, type A behavior, irritable mood, demoralization) represent an innovative instrument with therapeutic implications. When alexithymia is diagnosed, greater efforts will be made to increase the patients' awareness of the emotions underlying disordered eating behaviors. Moreover, in a comprehensive intervention, the diagnosis of demoralization and irritable mood increases the therapist's understanding of the patients' cognitive and relational patterns and suggests the use of an antidepressant. Alexithymia and type A behavior describe more stable traits in relation with the patients' personality. From this viewpoint, psychotherapy may be focused on the identification and expression of feelings, giving particular attention to anger, which is often unrecognized, excessively controlled, and self-destructive in patients with EDs. Lastly, the correlation between personality traits assessed with the Temperament and Character Inventory and the Diagnostic Criteria for Psychosomatic Research suggests that the strengthening of character through psychodynamic psychotherapy might be useful also for the psychosomatic cores of the disorder.

Eating disorders (EDs) are widespread in Western society and their incidence has increased throughout the last decade in the 'at-risk' population [1]. Although the best known clinical pictures are anorexia nervosa (AN) and bulimia nervosa (BN), about 50% of the patients applying to specialized units suffer from EDs not otherwise specified. The EDs not otherwise specified include subthreshold EDs and binge eating disorder (BED) and share chronicity and severity with full-syndrome EDs [2, 3]. The social ramifications of EDs also include the high cost of treatment [4], which is similar to that of the most severe psychiatric disorders [5]. In addition, inadequate treatment can lead to an overall increase in the social and health costs of EDs [6, 7].

EDs have a complex pathogenesis and several predisposing and perpetuating biopsychosocial factors [8]. The role of some psychological aspects is relevant for clinical practice but still must be defined. Specifically, the psychosomatic mechanisms underlying EDs have been acknowledged for a long time, but their role still needs to be clarified with regard to treatment.

EDs have been classically considered psychosomatic disorders [9, 10] for several reasons:

1. These disorders express themselves through behaviors aimed at controlling one's body, but at the same time they also suggest the loss of control over it. Psychological suffering is expressed through somatic suffering until it becomes 'a language which is more expressive than words: the language of organs' [11]. In EDs the psychosomatic and somatopsychic unity of the individual becomes extremely clear.
2. Once the disorder is clear, a vicious cycle begins, both from biopsychic and psychobiologic viewpoints, which perpetuates the disorder through a severe neuroendocrine deregulation. The activation of the hypothalamic-pituitary-adrenal axis, the decrease of gonadal hormones, and the involvement of the hypothalamic centers regulating hunger and satiety are widely acknowledged [12]. Recently, the stressing role of these systems on the brain has been underscored [13]. Furthermore, the alterations caused by starvation lead to (or increase) mood instability, obsessiveness, insomnia, and hyperactivity [14]. Finally, the progress in biomedical techniques in the last 15 years has allowed the identification of some relevant neuromodulators in AN and BN, for example the alteration in the levels of ghrelin [15], which affects hunger/satiety and also psychical symptoms [16].
3. In EDs, the difficulty of recognizing and expressing one's emotions is widely acknowledged [17, 18] and is a typical alexithymic feature. This difficulty makes the individuals confused in their ability to discriminate their psychological and somatic needs (e.g. frustration versus hunger). The psychosomatic issues and their relationships with the developing identity, the problems concerning separation, and the relationship with one's mother represent the core elements of the 'disperceptive' theories of EDs.
4. The communication patterns within the family represent another core issue of EDs [19–22] and are typically confused and distorted. Minuchin et al. [23] described the anorectic family as 'psychosomatic family'; among family members there is an excessive involvement with difficulties in

defining the generational and personal boundaries. Every member of the family is excessively involved with the other ones, nobody is able to assert his/her own needs, and everyone tends to speak for the others, with an overall loss of one's sense of identity. These concepts have been developed also for the other EDs.

Currently, the new psychosomatic medicine refers to the aforesaid ideas and supports a modern comprehensive concept of medicine [24]. Three issues have been underscored: (1) the role of psychosocial factors as a cause of vulnerability, (2) the interaction of psychosocial and biologic factors on the course of the disorder, and (3) the use of psychological therapies in prevention and treatment.

Evidence-based medicine must verify the theoretical issues that suggest a relationship between EDs and psychosomatic disorders.

Since the 1970s, the scientific community has investigated the relationship between EDs and psychosomatic issues, with a constant and progressive interest. A PubMed search gives more than 400 results for studies (in English) about the empirical investigation of the relationship between eating-disordered attitudes and psychosomatic medicine. The theories mentioned above are supported by data that can be summed up in five major research trends:

1. New findings concerning the endocrine, metabolic, and brain mechanisms related to EDs.
2. Pathogenic and predisposing role of psychosomatic traits in EDs.
3. Relationship among emotions, difficulties in their identification and management, and tendency to eat too much or too little.
4. Relationship between psychosomatic cores and eating psychopathology.
5. Treatment focused on psychosomatic issues.

Psychological Antecedents

Risk factors and early life events in EDs represent predisposing/vulnerability factors and are partly mediated by the typical psychosomatic mechanisms, including both the psycho-neuro-endocrine system (early stressing events, not acute/chronic ones) and the development of personality traits or of specific ways of coping with emotions. The literature about the risk factors for EDs is abundant and a detailed description is beyond the scope of this chapter. A recent and exhaustive review provides a deeper understanding of this subject [25].

Briefly, the research areas that have been developed to date are:

1. Perinatal stressing events: role of obstetric complications [26], of low weight as a consequence of premature birth [27], period of birth [28].

2. Disturbed family relations during childhood, parents' general and eating psychopathology (these issues are discussed in the chapter).
3. Role of adverse experiences, in particular the controversial traumatic role of sexual abuse, which is sometimes thought to have a specific pathogenic role [29], though there is no agreement about its specificity [30].
4. Role of the life events preceding the onset of the disorder, which have been recently suggested to be something more than simple 'trigger events.' Familiar conflict, change of residence, change of school have been found to precede the onset of EDs [31, 32]. Severe stressing events are thought to increase significantly the risk of developing anorexia or bulimia [33]. The early phase of bulimia is characterized by a prodrome of depressive symptoms and stressful life events [34]. The only study about BED [35] has found many stressful life events (including critical comments about shape and weight, work-related stress, major changes in life, etc.) in the year before the onset of the disorder.

A careful anamnesis can allow the identification of these constellations of adverse life events during different phases of one's life. The data collected through the anamnesis are useful for the clinician to identify the possible pathogenesis of the patient's disorder, with a comprehensive psychosomatic perspective. Furthermore, the significant life events allow an understanding of the subject's conscious and unconscious background, which is an important requirement for the engagement of patients with EDs.

Psychological Aspects

Psychiatric Comorbidity

The comorbidity of EDs and other axis I and axis II psychiatric diagnoses is high and represents a difficulty in the treatment of these disorders. Data suggest a lifetime comorbidity rate of 50–60%; personality disorders (PDs) are found in the 70% of patients. Only 20% of patients do not receive other diagnoses along time [36]. Anxiety and depressive disorders are the more common ones. With more detail, depression and obsessive-compulsive disorder are the more frequent comorbid disorders in anorexia and bulimia. A substance use disorder is often found in purging subjects. As regards PDs, AN and BED are frequently comorbid with cluster C disorders, while BN with cluster B disorders [37]. BED is characterized by a higher rate of comorbid depressive disorder [38]. A more thorough description of this issue is beyond the aim of this chapter; more details about the prevalence of comorbid disorders in EDs and treatment can be found in some systematic reviews [39–42].

Psychosomatic Comorbidity (Pilot Study)

As described in the conceptual issues chapter by Fabbri et al. [pp. 1–20], a new research instrument has been proposed to make the concepts used in psychosomatics clearer and more measurable. The diagnostic criteria proposed by the authors represent practical guidelines for the identification of those psychological factors that are relevant for clinical practice and that can be considered as adjuncts to axis I and axis II diagnoses and medical conditions.

The Diagnostic Criteria for Psychosomatic Research (DCPR) have been used in patients with gastroenteric, cardiac, dermatologic, endocrine, and neoplastic disorders, in patients with somatoform disorders, and in liaison psychiatry, as described by others [43–52]. The DCPR proved useful in confirming diagnoses, assessing psychological factors that worsen the quality of life, verifying some classical psychosomatic theories, identifying at-risk groups of patients, and predicting outcome. In the general population (347 subjects), the finding of alexithymia, type A behavior, and irritable mood is quite common and correlates with a worse quality of life [53].

Currently, there are no studies about the use of DCPR in EDs, though the psychosomatic core of anorexia and bulimia has been widely demonstrated and acknowledged, as described in the previous paragraphs.

A pilot study by the EDs Centre of Turin University has used the DCPR in patients with AN, BN, and BED. We used the four diagnostic categories in the area of 'psychological factors influencing illness vulnerability'. It is likely that the areas 'abnormal illness behavior' and 'somatization' are influenced by the psychosomatic alterations that are consequent to the extreme weight fluctuations typical of EDs, so it would be better to assess these areas after remission.

The aim of the study was to:

- apply for the first time the diagnostic criteria for research in psychosomatics (DCPR) in patients with EDs;
- compare patients with a psychosomatic diagnosis with those with no psychosomatic diagnosis in the following variables: eating psychopathology, anger levels, depressive symptoms, and personality;
- identify the correlation among psychosomatic diagnoses, eating psychopathology, anger levels, depressive symptoms, and personality.

We assessed 102 consecutive patients in the outpatient service of our ED Centre in the last 6 months of 2005. We excluded from the study only those subjects with a lifetime history of psychosis (3 subjects). All the patients were assessed by psychiatrists with the Structured Clinical Interview for DSM-IV. The same psychiatrist assessed the patients with the DCPR during the three evaluation sessions, which are proposed to all the patients applying to our ED Centre. During this phase, all the patients completed the following

Table 1. Sample characteristics

	BN	ANR	ANBP	NOS	BED
Patients	11	37	14	30	10
Age	28.1 ± 9.82	24.18 ± 7.61	25.32 ± 6.49	23.90 ± 6.01	36.14 ± 8.42
BMI	21.15 ± 1.49	14.17 ± 0.94	16.12 ± 1.78	19.31 ± 0.71	25.83 ± 3.43
Schooling	11.40 ± 1.84	11.12 ± 2.05	12.29 ± 2.09	19.32 ± 0.74	10.97 ± 2.24

NOS = Not otherwise specified; BMI = body mass index.

Table 2. Total sample

	Alexithymia	Type A behavior	Demoralization	Irritable mood
BN	6 (54%)	4 (36%)	6 (54%)	6 (54%)
ANR	25 (68%)	24 (38%)	27 (73%)	7 (19%)
ANBP	3 (21%)	2 (14%)	7 (50%)	12 (86%)
NOS	13 (43)%	5 (17%)	6 (20%)	11 (37%)
BED	66 (0%)	22 (0%)	3 (30%)	5 (50%)
Total	53 (52%)	27 (27%)	49 (48%)	41 (40%)

self-administered questionnaires: the Temperament and Character Inventory (TCI) [54] for the assessment of personality; the Eating Disorder Inventory-2 (EDI-2) [55] for eating psychopathology; the State and Trait Anger Expression Inventory (STAXI) [56] for anger, and the Beck Depression Inventory (BDI) [57] for the assessment of depressive symptoms.

The subdivision of the sample and its features are reported in table 1. Alexithymia was found in 52% of the whole sample, type A behaviors in 27% of subjects, demoralization in 48%, and irritable mood in 40% of patients. The rates found in the different diagnostic categories are reported in table 2. Overall, patients with restrictor anorexia have the higher rates of alexithymia, type A behavior, and demoralization, but lower rates of irritable mood.

Patients matching the diagnostic criteria for each of the four categories were compared to the patients who did not match the criteria. The mean scores on the TCI, STAXI, EDI-2, and BDI were compared with the t test for independent samples. An $\alpha \leq 0.05$ was considered statistically significant.

Patients matching the diagnostic criteria for alexithymia had lower Novelty seeking and Self-directedness on the TCI; they had higher scores on the

Table 3. Alexithymia

	Alexithymia (n = 53)	No diagnosis of alexithymia (n = 49)	t	p
TCI NS	17.04 ± 5.58	21.63 ± 6.52	3.76	0.001
TCI SD	24.04 ± 8.70	18.03 ± 7.39	5.67	0.001
EDI-2 ID	8.14 ± 4.76	6.00 ± 4.51	−2.27	0.025
EDI-2 SI	9.56 ± 5.45	7.48 ± 3.85	−2.17	0.032

TCI NS = TCI Novelty seeking; TCI SD = TCI Self-directedness; EDI-2 ID = EDI-2 Interpersonal distrust; EDI-2 SI = EDI-2 Social insecurity.

Table 4. Type A behavior

	Type A behavior (n = 27)	No diagnosis of type A behavior (n = 75)	t	p
TCI P	573 ± 1.37	4.86 ± 2.04	−2.00	0.048
TCI C	32.65 ± 6.33	29.41 ± 8.71	−2.02	0.048
TCI ST	16.15 ± 6.92	12.68 ± 6.08	−2.26	0.029
STAXI S-Ang	11.54 ± 2.26	15.48 ± 6.73	2.91	0.004
STAXI AX/IN	17.69 ± 4.15	20.11 ± 5.43	2.05	0.042
STAXI AX/EX	28.38 ± 9.81	33.25 ± 11.42	2.07	0.044

TCI P = TCI Persistence; TCI C = TCI Cooperativeness; TCI ST = TCI Self-transcendence; STAXI S-Ang = STAXI State-anger; STAXI AX/IN = STAXI Anger-in; STAXI AX/EX = STAXI Anger expression.

Interpersonal distrust and Social insecurity scales of the EDI-2, whereas no difference emerged in the anger levels and depressive symptoms between the two groups (table 3).

Patients matching the diagnostic criteria for type A behavior had higher Persistence, Cooperativeness, and Self-transcendence on the TCI; they had lower scores on state anger, introverted (Anger in), and overall anger, whereas no difference emerged in eating psychopathology and depression symptoms (table 4).

Patients matching the diagnostic criteria for demoralization scored significantly lower on the TCI scale of Self-directedness; they scored higher on temperamental anger and extroverted anger on the STAXI; they had higher

Table 5. Demoralization

	Demoralization (n = 49)	No diagnosis of demoralization (n = 53)	t	p
TCI SD	19.35 ± 8.92	23.04 ± 8.88	2.06	0.042
STAXI T-Ang	22.92 ± 5.93	19.57 ± 4.41	−3.14	0.002
STAXI T-Ang/T	8.00 ± 3.17	6.33 ± 1.90	−3.13	0.002
STAXI T-Ang/R	11.04 ± 3.13	9.63 ± 2.76	−2.34	0.021
EDI-2 IN	13.79 ± 7.74	8.31 ± 6.17	−3.84	0.001
EDI-2 PERF	6.38 ± 4.03	4.65 ± 4.26	−2.06	0.041
EDI-2 ID	8.47 ± 4.99	5.82 ± 4.17	−2.83	0.006
EDI-2 MF	8.57 ± 5.04	5.55 ± 5.07	−2.83	0.006
EDI-2 ASC	8.53 ± 5.06	5.98 ± 3.58	−2.85	0.005
EDI-2 IMPUL	9.62 ± 6.61	5.37 ± 5.59	−3.41	0.001
EDI-2 SI	10.45 ± 5.03	6.78 ± 3.92	−3.99	0.001
BDI	17.52 ± 7.58	11.69 ± 7.70	−3.67	0.001

TCI SD = TCI Self-directedness; STAXI T-Ang = STAXI Trait Anger; STAXI T-Ang/T = STAXI Trait Angry temperament; STAXI T-Ang/R = STAXI Trait Angry reaction; EDI-2 IN = EDI-2 Ineffectiveness; EDI-2 PERF = EDI-2 Perfectionism; EDI-2 ID = EDI-2 Interpersonal distrust; EDI-2 MF = EDI-2 Maturity fears; EDI-2 ASC = EDI-2 Asceticism; EDI-2 IMPUL = EDI-2 Impulse regulation; EDI-2 SI = EDI-2 Social insecurity.

Ineffectiveness, Perfectionism, Interpersonal distrust, Maturity fears, Asceticism, Impulsiveness, and Social insecurity on the EDI-2, and higher levels of depression on the BDI (table 5).

Patients matching criteria for irritable mood scored lower on Self-directedness and Cooperativeness on the TCI; they had higher state anger, trait anger, extroverted anger (Anger out), and overall anger on the STAXI and a lower control of anger (Anger control). Moreover, they scored higher on the EDI-2 subscales of Bulimia, Ineffectiveness, Asceticism, Impulsiveness, and Social insecurity, and on the BDI (table 6).

The amount of preliminary data leads to several clinical considerations, which can be useful hints for future research about psychosomatic diagnoses and EDs.

According to the findings that emerged with the use of DCPR, psychosomatic diagnoses are frequently found in EDs, supporting the relationship among disordered eating attitudes and psychosomatics described in the literature by studies using mainly self-administered questionnaires [58–66]. Among the diagnostic categories of EDs, the restrictor subtype of AN (ANR) is the one with higher rates of psychosomatic traits according to the DCPR. This can be

Table 6. Irritable mood

	Irritable mood (n = 41)	No diagnosis of irritable mood (n = 61)	t	p
TCI SD	17.69 ± 8.94	23.57 ± 8.41	3.26	0.002
TCI C	27.21 ± 10.06	32.25 ± 6.13	2.81	0.007
STAXI S-Ang	16.13 ± 7.98	13.32 ± 4.22	−1.99	0.050
STAXI T-Ang	23.47 ± 5.96	19.78 ± 4.60	−3.24	0.002
STAXI T-Ang/T	8.11 ± 2.98	6.54 ± 2.38	−2.71	0.008
STAXI AX-OUT	17.89 ± 5.43	15.25 ± 6.24	−2.13	0.035
STAXI AX-CON	18.47 ± 6.17	21.05 ± 6.08	2.02	0.047
STAXI AX-EX	37.05 ± 12.50	28.66 ± 8.88	−3.59	0.001
EDI 2-BU	8.00 ± 7.32	5.17 ± 5.19	−2.07	0.042
EDI 2-IN	13.21 ± 7.33	9.50 ± 7.23	−2.46	0.016
EDI 2-ASC	8.47 ± 4.72	6.40 ± 4.22	−2.20	0.031
EDI 2-IMPUL	10.24 ± 6.67	5.62 ± 5.63	−3.54	0.001
EDI 2-SI	10.37 ± 4.02	7.38 ± 5.45	−2.91	0.005
BDI	17.71 ± 8.32	13.28 ± 7.85	−1.98	0.049

TCI SD = TCI Self-directedness; TCI C = TCI cooperativeness; STAXI S-Ang = STAXI State Anger; STAXI T-Ang = STAXI Trait Anger; STAXI T-Ang/T = STAXI Trait Angry temperament; STAXI AX-OUT = STAXI Anger-out; STAXI AX-CON = STAXI Anger control; STAXI AX-EX = STAXI Anger expression; EDI-2 BU = EDI-2 Bulimia; EDI-2 IN = EDI-2 Ineffectiveness; EDI-2 ASC = EDI-2 Asceticism; EDI-2 IMPUL = EDI-2 Impulse regulation; EDI 2 SI = EDI 2 Social insecurity.

the consequence of the personality features of these patients (rigidity and difficulty in recognizing emotions) but also of the severe somatic alterations typical of these patients. Moreover, considering the distribution of diagnoses, two different patterns seem to emerge. The first is typical of patients with a tendency to overcontrol (ANR) and the second is typical of patients with a tendency to lose control (BN, AN-binge/purging, BED, and not otherwise specified). The first group of patients is characterized by more marked alexithymic traits, rigidity, control over aggressive feelings, and depression. Patients belonging to the second group are more impulsive and angry (high rates of irritable mood). The DCPR seem to support the different patterns of coping with impulses (e.g. anger) [67] but also the psychosomatic differences between AN and BN [68]. Patients with ANBP anorexia share features with bulimic patients, but not with patients with restrictor AN. The fact that ANBP and BN share personality features has already been suggested and supported [69].

Considering the four diagnoses in the area 'psychological factors influencing illness vulnerability' and their relation with personality and symptoms, in

EDs there is a poor correlation among alexithymia and type A behavior, on one side, and eating symptoms and depression, on the other. They seem to be more stable traits underlying the disorder, and these psychosomatic features are shared by many patients. Instead, irritable mood and demoralization have several correlations with eating symptoms and depression and seem more related to the illness or directly to symptoms. They are more simple concepts that can be shared by different personality types.

As far as the alexithymic personality is concerned, irritable mood and demoralization correlate with more fragile and immature character traits, whereas type A behavior correlates with a more controlling and rigid personality. The temperamental traits of personality correlate with the more complex psychosomatic issues as alexithymia and type A behavior. On the other hand, character traits have more widespread and relevant correlation with the psychosomatic diagnoses, particularly Self-directedness, as already suggested by other authors [70, 71]. Moreover, depressive symptoms do not correlate in a linear way with alexithymia and type A behavior, supporting the existence of a partial relationship, but not of interdependence, among these traits.

For the correlation among DCPR and STAXI scores, the correlation among anger management (i.e. identification, expression, and suppression of angry feelings) and psychosomatic diagnoses suggested by theoretical models [72] is supported. Patients with type A behavior tend to deny hostility on the STAXI. Lastly, the strong correlation between the 'irritable mood' diagnosis and the STAXI supports the reliability of the concepts underlying the diagnostic criterion identified by the clinician. A diagnosis that allows the identification of anger is clearly useful for clinical psychiatrists.

These data are still preliminary and further research is needed. The small size of the sample does not allow us to perform a multivariate analysis of data, which limits the impact of the conclusions. The several and relevant correlations among DCPR and EDs support the clinical importance of the new diagnoses. It clearly emerges that at least half of the patients with EDs have a relevant psychosomatic core, whereas for other patients this is not so important. The therapeutic implications are discussed in the following paragraphs.

Discussion of Hostility, Irritable Mood, Alexithymia, Demoralization and Type A Behavior

Negative Emotions, Anger, Irritable Mood and Eating Disorders

It is widely acknowledged that conscious and unconscious negative emotions (sadness, anxiety, feelings of emptiness and loneliness, weariness, frustration, anger, etc.) can lead to disordered eating patterns, which can represent the prodrome of a disorder as well as symptoms of the disorder itself. An unsuited management of negative emotions, characterized by ineffective mechanisms of suppression, repression, and ineffective elaboration through mature defenses (e.g. rationalization, tolerance of frustration, ability to think about emotions) is typical of psychosomatic disorders and is related to EDs. An interesting description of the theoretical models is provided by Canetti et al. [73]. Anger is one of the most important among negative emotions because of its malignant implications as well as its clinical relevance for the treatment of EDs (anger and impulsiveness management).

Anger is a transnosographic dimension (mood, anxiety, PDs, etc.). Anger, hostility, and irritability are psychopathologic elements that often require a pressing and specific intervention [74], and this is particularly true when these elements are hidden or unconscious, as they often are in EDs. Aggressiveness and anger, especially self-directed, are common in all EDs [75]. Particularly, in BN the expression/suppression of anger has been related to the specific core beliefs of the disorder [76]. Recently, a study of 190 obese patients [77] showed that angry feelings are the only element shared by both men and women and predicts a disordered eating style. The authors state that anger management is an important objective in the treatment of these patients. Fassino et al. [78] showed that impulsive anger is more common in BED obese patients than in obese patients without BED; the latter tend to suppress anger. Another recent study supports the role of anger as a negative emotion that frequently leads to binges [79].

In AN, the unconscious feeling of self-worthlessness leads patients to negative emotions and anger, which are maintaining factors of the disorder, together with a difficulty in controlling impulses. In BN and BED, there is a more conscious anguish of being abandoned, which stimulates an unconscious anger toward parents and masochistic behaviors of destruction/reparation. From this viewpoint, intake and expulsion of food represent a perverse aggression against one's body [80, 81]. In all EDs, impulsiveness, aggressiveness, and anger are relevant psychopathologic elements [82, 83]. In BN, stronger angry feelings correlate with suicide attempts [84] and also with the frequency of vomiting [85]. In all EDs, laxative abuse correlates with anger, impulsiveness, and borderline personality traits [86]. Patients with EDs have high degrees of self-criticism and their EDs may be an angry protest against an external authority [87], with different patterns in men and women with BN [88]. Impulsiveness and acting out can correlate with the difficulty of expressing aggressive feelings [83] and with the personality features typical of psychosomatic disorders [21, 22, 89].

Hostility, poor tolerance of frustration, and aggressiveness in patients with EDs represent a way of entering into relationships with other people that is partly influenced by warped family relationships [90] and childhood experiences [81, 91, 92]. Bulimic patients are more impulsive than anorectic ones and those bulimics with lower degrees of impulsiveness have a faster response to treatment [93], but also more frequent relapses. There are hypotheses concerning an alteration of the serotonin system [94, 95], given the high incidence of aggressive attitudes and behaviors, also against the therapist (though often indirectly), and given the typical difficulty in the control of impulses of EDs. Some authors [96] have found that anger attacks are more common in bulimic patients than in a control group. For these reasons, patients with EDs can lead therapists to 'burnout' because of aggressive and angry feelings, which are indirectly expressed by anorectics (e.g. weight loss) or directly by bulimics (e.g. acting out).

Studies performed by the Centre for the Diagnosis and Treatment of Eating Disorders of Turin University [97] showed that different patterns of anger management exist in bulimic and anorectic patients and that these patterns influence the response to treatment. Patients with BN have higher degrees of temperamental anger and tend to feel angry when they are undervalued or when their self-esteem is under attack. Bulimic patients tend to express their anger in an impulsive way, both against things and people. Furthermore, bulimic patients have a low tolerance for frustrations, whereas anorectic individuals have a pathologic high tolerance for frustration and devaluation.

The anorectic patient tends to deny angry feelings and to suppress them, so that the anger levels are not much different from those of a control subject. Bulimic patients, on the other hand, manage and express their angry feelings in a more sensational way. Bulimic patients are extra-punitive, whereas anorectics are intra-punitive.

To be true, these two different ways of managing angry feelings represent the reverse sides of the same coin and are both 'immature.' Bulimic behaviors have been correlated with angry feelings, particularly with state anger, that is, with the anger related to specific situations. The association of anger and behaviors like vomiting or laxative abuse depends mainly on the baseline personality of the subject, which conditions the emotional reactions to intrapsychic and relational conflicts. Patients with a less adaptive and more 'immature' character (low Self-directedness on the TCI) are at greater risk of self-aggressive behaviors, independently of the ED diagnosis. Moreover, in regard to temperament, the excessive expression of anger and anger suppression correlate with the two dimensions of Novelty seeking and Harm avoidance, respectively.

Patients with a character profile as the one described above are more impulsive and angry and are at greater risk of having a PD [98].

The study of anger and personality traits in EDs gave interesting results with regard to the response to and compliance with treatment. It is widely acknowledged that many patients with EDs (up to the 50%) drop out from treatment early, especially psychotherapies, although they consistently attend nutritional and endocrinology outpatient services. Many patients prefer a treatment approach focused on the body, which does not represent a menace for their defensive structure and allows the maintenance of a 'safer' situation, just as occurs for psychosomatic patients.

It has been demonstrated that the lack of an at least partial awareness of the dynamics underlying the ED predicts a negative prognosis [99, 100] and a greater risk of relapse.

The study of dropout from psychotherapy is relevant to plan treatment interventions in public facilities and to understand and modify those factors related to treatment compliance. Some specific character dimensions, such as low Self-directedness and Cooperativeness measured with the TCI, are relevant risk factors for an early dropout from brief psychotherapy [101]. Also in this case, those patients who give up treatment are angrier and have a greater difficulty recognizing and coping with aggressive feelings, which seems to depend on disturbed and disturbing character traits.

Although several studies investigated the relationships among emotions, eating, and eating psychopathology, all these issues have been studied mainly with self-administered questionnaires, which are at risk of overestimation [102] and do not allow a clear distinction between normality and pathology.

The introduction of specific diagnostic criteria for relevant issues as 'irritable mood' and 'demoralization' [103] opens a new, clinically based perspective, in the context of a wider scientific and cultural proposal concerning a new approach to the DSM axis system. 'Back to clinical medicine' is the main concept of this modern approach [104].

Alexithymia

Alexithymia is the most debated issue concerning the relationship between psychosomatics and EDs. A PubMed search yields more than 100 studies about this subject (studies and reviews). Many authors agree that patients with AN and BN show alexithymic traits more frequently than healthy controls [58–66]. A study about enteroceptive awareness performed on 173 patients with EDs and 49 obese patients found that all the patients, mostly bulimic ones, reported difficulties in discriminating sensations, feelings, and hunger/satiety. Alexithymic traits were predicted by depression, perfectionism, and a poorly self-directive personality [105].

Alexithymic traits were found in EDs more frequently than in other psychiatric disorders [106], but the literature on this subject is still scarce and further research is needed. Some recent studies found that alexithymic traits partly or totally persist when accounting for relevant confounding variables such as depressive symptoms [61, 64, 66], patient age, and illness duration [60] but not when accounting for negative affect, which is the core of alexithymia itself [107]. In any case, these data show the stability of alexithymic traits in anorexia and bulimia, supporting their pathogenic role. Alexithymia is related to the eating restrictions and anger suppression [108] typical of these patients [109]. Furthermore, it is related to the avoiding PD both in AN and BN and, though less frequently, to other PDs [60] typically comorbid with EDs [36]. Finally, the emotional disorders of anorectic and bulimic patients worsen their performance on neuropsychological tests [110], except for purely cognitive tests [111]. The alteration of neuropsychological tests is typical of ED patients and it correlates with the body image disorder in AN [112].

The differences between anorectic and bulimic patients in regard to alexithymia have not been thoroughly investigated and the existing data are controversial [61, 63, 68].

Alexithymia has been studied also in the families of ED patients. Two studies describe the possible role of parents in alexithymia. The parents of 43 anorectic patients and of 30 bulimics scored higher on the Toronto Alexithymia Scale (TAS-20) than the 72 parents of healthy controls [113]. Furthermore, a poor level of maternal care during childhood, measured with the Parental Bonding Instrument, correlated with high scores on the TAS-20 in 68 ED patients [114].

Recently, attention has been paid also to alexithymia and BED. A generic relation exists between alexithymia and obesity [115, 116], but alexithymic traits and psychosomatic issues are more specifically correlated to BED than to overweight [117–120]. Furthermore, the higher the scores on the Binge Eating Scale, the higher are those on the subscale of the TAS-20 describing the difficulties in recognizing and describing feelings [121].

As already underscored for 'irritable mood' and 'demoralization,' the introduction of categorical diagnostic criteria for alexithymia [104] may allow for more careful research on these traits and their role in EDs.

Type A Behavior

The type A behavior has been widely studied as a possible risk factor in the field of cardiovascular disease [122]. This is a complex concept related to some personality traits, but the literature concerning this issue in psychiatric disorders is still scarce, perhaps because of its complex overlapping with axis I and axis II diagnoses [123].

There are reasons supporting the importance of studying the type A behavior in EDs, and particularly in AN, given the typical dynamics of this disorder, with control, competition, and perfectionism representing specific risk factors [124]. There is only one study in the literature about this subject;

Brunner et al. [125] found type A behavior to be more common in anorectics and in weight-recovered anorectics than in controls. Also in patients with AN, these aggressive traits correlate with the cardiovascular function. The introduction of diagnostic criteria for type A behavior may provide avenues for future research.

Personality: Temperament, Character, Eating Disorders, and Psychosomatic Issues

Alexithymia is a complex concept describing a specific way of thinking, feeling, and behaving; this is the reason authors have described an alexithymic personality since the beginning [126]. In the last 30 years, this issue has been widely debated and sometimes criticized, according to the relationship between alexithymia and other psychopathologic elements. Moreover, some authors have argued about the stability of the traits described as 'alexithymic.' The concept of alexithymic personality seems to have an undoubted clinical relevance, and it has recently been related to other personality features, proving stable in repeated tests [70, 127]. The study of personality in psychiatry and in psychosomatics is relevant because it allows for a better understanding of the patient and a more careful planning of treatment, and it may also be a predictor of the response to treatment. The DSM-IV-TR diagnostic criteria include those for PDs [99], but exclude some significant traits such as the alexithymic ones.

For EDs, the study of personality is fundamental, too. The complexity of EDs led the authors to two different approaches in the study of personality. The first approach is the categorical one, that is, the axis II diagnosis of a PD. A comorbid PD in an ED patient may influence the course of the disorder, treatment outcome [99], and the clinical picture of the ED itself [128, 129]. The second approach is the dimensional one, that is, the identification of a baseline personality profile, which increases the subject's risk of developing an ED [98].

The categorical approach found a prevalence of cluster C PDs ranging from 0 to 22% [130, 131] in AN and of cluster B PDs ranging from 2 to 50% in BN [36, 132, 133]. For the dimensional approach, several authors investigated the temperament and character dimensions with the Tridimensional Personality Questionnaire and the TCI developed by Cloninger [134] and Svrakic et al. [135]. These questionnaires allowed the identification of some specific traits for AN and BN, and the study of the role of personality as regards the course, treatment, and prognosis of these disorders. Furthermore, the dimensional approach to the study of personality allows the integration of the biopsychosocial issues underlying psychiatric disorders, because it considers the genetic-biologic issues and their relation with the dynamic-environmental ones.

The study of the personality dimensions of anorectic patients with the TCI made it possible to deepen the understanding of their personality traits and also to make neurophysiologic, therapeutic, and prognostic inferences related to their temperament and character [67, 109, 136, 137]. Anorectic patients are characterized by high Harm avoidance, low Novelty seeking, and high Reward dependence as regards temperament [138–143] and by low Self-directedness and high Persistence as regards character [144]. Bulimic patients score high on Harm avoidance, as anorectics [145], but they are different from anorectics because they have higher Novelty seeking [142] and Reward dependence [139] but lower Self-directedness [142, 146]. Binge-purging anorectics share some personality features with restrictor anorectics and others with bulimics [69]. More details concerning this issue can be found in a review we published a few years ago [147].

The TCI has also been used to study the correlations among alexithymic traits and temperament and character dimensions. Both temperament and character correlate with alexithymia; however, the studies with the TCI concerning this issue are still in their early phase.

Low scores on Reward dependence and Self-directedness and, to a lesser extent, high scores on Harm avoidance predict alexithymia in a sample of 254 outpatients [71], though they do not explain the whole variance. The TCI subscales seem to play a role, too. A similar study performed on 220 students with no psychiatric disorders supports these data. Furthermore, in the same study, low scores on Cooperativeness predict alexithymia [70]. Neuroimaging studies found a correlation among the volume of the right anterior cingulate gyrus, alexithymic traits, and Harm avoidance in healthy subjects, which was stronger in female subjects [148]. This result opens an interesting neurobiologic perspective about the concepts of personality and alexithymia, which deserves further investigation. Currently, the only clinical population investigated is that of drug addicts. Drug addicts with a history of attempted suicide score low on Self-directedness and cooperativeness and high on the TAS-20 [149]. In the same sample, self-mutilation behaviors correlated with high scores on alexithymia, with no significant result in regard to the TCI [150].

The limitation shared by these studies is the use of the TAS-20 for the assessment of alexithymic traits. The TAS-20 is widely used and studied, but remains a self-administered questionnaire with its typical limits. The proposal of specific diagnostic criteria for the diagnosis of alexithymia may support or not the findings of the studies performed to date. This objective is further discussed later in the chapter.

Treatment

The treatment of EDs is multimodal [100, 151]. The psychosomatic assessment of patients, together with the assessment of personality and of the motivation/resistance to treatment [69], are required to plan a multimodal treatment, which articulates in a noncontradictory way [152] drug therapy, individual and family psychotherapy, and diet therapy. The treatment of EDs is 'psychosomatic' because it requires the association of nutritional, psychiatric, and psychotherapeutic treatments, which strengthen each other [100].

The vicious psychosomatic and somatopsychic circle of severe malnutrition in anorexia, of the chaotic eating patterns of binges and purging behaviors, and of their association, is a perpetuating factor for EDs.

From this viewpoint, the identification of further specific psychosomatic diagnoses, as the DCPR proposed and previously discussed, allows an understanding of and change in the psychosomatic cores that underlie and perpetuate EDs.

The identification of negative emotions (irritable mood and demoralization), which are not recognized by patients and are not totally accounted for by the axis I psychiatric diagnoses, allows clinicians to work to increase the patients' enteroceptive awareness, according to the disperceptive theories. The objective is to help patients develop new coping strategies for stress and new ways of expressing their suffering, apart from food and body image.

In a more comprehensive perspective, there is the need to assess alexithymic traits and control patterns in patients with anorexia, bulimia and BED, and the 'alexithymia' and 'type A behavior' diagnoses fulfill this need. As some important authors suggested in a passionate paper about emotions and fantasy in EDs [58], at the beginning of psychotherapy and any kind of treatment, it is important to understand the patients' ability to recognize and express their emotions and feelings, the level of development of their ability in making fantasies, and their locus of control.

The study of interventions and of the prognostic role of alexithymic traits in EDs has just begun. The treatment approaches emphasizing the importance of identifying and expressing feelings and emotions are recommended [58], but the literature concerning this issue is too scarce. Beales and Dolton [153] found alexithymic traits in 72% of the patients during the acute phase of AN and in 33% during the remission phase. It is debated whether the improvement of anorexia includes the improvement of alexithymia or the absence of alexithymia makes remission from anorexia easier. A follow-up study reports an improvement of alexithymic traits at 1 year of follow-up after cognitive behavioral therapy (CBT) in bulimic patients [154], whereas Iancu et al. [65] recently found that the improvement of symptoms in EDs is not correlated with the changes in alexithymic traits. A psychodynamic study of the outcome of brief Adlerian psychodynamic psychotherapy with the Karolinska Personality Profile found that the improvement of alexithymic traits in anorectic and bulimic patients correlates with a better compliance with treatment and with the improvement of symptoms, and that those patients with more marked alexithymic traits are more likely to have a poor response to treatment [155].

The treatment of EDs includes: (1) psychopharmacologic treatments according to the guidelines and to the evidence reported by randomized, controlled trials and (2) psychodynamic psychotherapy alternating supportive and intensive-expressive interventions [151, 156, 157]. As regards psychotherapy, CBT proved effective in the treatment of BN. Some authors used CBT also in AN and Interpersonal Psychotherapy was used in EDs as well. Some studies suggest that the latter is lower than CBT in changing the symptoms of EDs. More details about the psychotherapic treatment of EDs can be found in some systematic reviews [158–162]. Here follows the description of some issues of dynamic psychotherapy.

The treatment of EDs is often planned as a stepped-care approach [163], according to the model of sequential treatment [164]. The main feature of the treatment of EDs is the personalization of the therapeutic strategy depending on the need of modifying temperamental and character traits [165]. 'Strategy' refers to the planning of a project, usually an outpatient treatment, but also day hospital or inpatient treatment, developed after an overall psychiatric and medical assessment, accounting also for DCPR.

The nature of the disorder in AN, BN, and BED makes patients look for treatment only after several years of illness, because ED symptoms and their effects on the body and on emotions have a deep self-protective meaning [155]. As a consequence, the symptoms of EDs tend to maintain and strengthen themselves, and they often become untreatable, chronic, and inaccessible to treatment [166]. Patients are willing to give up these mechanisms of self-defense only if they receive an equivalent 'emotional supply of love and tenderness' [167].

In AN, BN, and BED, action is important and the somatic issues are more important than the intrapsychic conflict (typical of the neurotic area), as an attempt to conciliate the need of dependence and the feelings of menace [168].

The strategy in EDs mostly depends on the degree of malnutrition and psychosomatic impairment of patients, and on the cooperation among them, their family, and therapists. The treatment of EDs is articulated in phases and alternates supportive and intensive interventions. The expressive-supportive psychotherapy is the core of treatment [169, 170]. The alternation of supportive and intensive phases seems to be the typical feature of the clinical strategy for patients with EDs, especially for those with a severe medical impairment. This alternation is not always predictable in the different phases of treatment.

Supportive Interventions

The supportive interventions are typical of the early phases of treatment and their aim is to stop the acute emergency and urgency situations, to start the psychopharmacologic and nutritional treatment, and to build the therapeutic 'net' [147]. The somatopsychic regression of the patients' self needs to be arrested and their own and their family's anguish and destructive issues need to be addressed. The patients' cooperation is crucial for this kind of intervention. The involvement of the family is another relevant supportive issue, and the younger the patient is and the less chronic is his/her disorder, the more important is the involvement of family [20, 171, 172]. The family is relevant with regard to the real positive or negative issues of their existential situation ('designed patients' according to Selvini-Palazzoli or Minuchin). The family can play a crucial role either as a support or as an obstacle to therapy, depending on how much the family colludes with the patient and on how the family responds to the patient's split and projected needs.

The parents of EDs patients often show alterations in personality [21, 172, 173]. These specific temperamental and character dimensions can be the focus of therapeutic interventions, both in individual counseling and group efforts. Parents sometimes ask for a psychotherapeutic intervention at later times.

The most studied approach for family treatment is the multifactor family therapy developed at the Maudsley Hospital of London [20, 174]. This approach considers the symptoms of EDs as the result of a complex interaction of etiologic factors and the communication and relational patterns within the family as a consequence of the disorder. The family is considered a significant resource for this kind of treatment and is involved in the eating re-education of patients [175].

Expressive Psychotherapeutic Interventions

Supportive interventions can be followed or associated with analytic-expressive phases. The relational issues are deepened during the expressive phases and the work on the therapeutic relationship has great importance, especially in cases of dependent and hostile transfers. In patients with AN, as regards 20-session psychotherapeutic interventions, the nonspecific supportive clinical management was superior to interpersonal psychotherapy, whereas CBT was intermediate [176]; on the other hand, the psychoanalytic therapy, together with the family therapy, seems to be the most effective among the psychotherapeutic interventions lasting at least 1 year [177]. When the patient's condition improves, the therapy can be intensified with the analysis of the lifestyle to better understand the patient's personality patterns [178].

Some Adlerian therapists [147, 155, 178] underscore the importance of unmasking the fictional goals that support the maladaptive behaviors of patients with AN. Food is considered a means to gain control over one's life, which the patient feels is difficult to rule as a consequence of deep feelings of self-worthlessness. This behavior gives patients a new (pathologic) identity that can be used as a means to avenge themselves, to pursue the fictional goal of perfection [179], and to hide feelings of emptiness and solitude. In its last phases, psychotherapy will encourage the rearrangement of Striving for power, the development of Social interest, and the use of cognitive skills and of the creative self to 'think and act as if she were the person she wanted to be' [180].

In BN and BED [181], it is necessary to focus on the dynamics of control and to underscore the emotional distance among the patient and the other people in the common situations of life. From a cognitive perspective, the all-or-nothing thinking is analyzed. A greater trust in one's own choices may allow new experiences and, in the long term, change the rigidity of thought. Patients can be further helped in correlating their mental perceptive scheme to their emotions and the ED [182]. This allows patients to understand that their behavior, according to a private logic, limits their functioning. From this point of view, the DCPR are a reliable instrument for the therapist's orientation.

In fact, the pathologic defenses are strengthened by the psychosomatic issues.

Conclusions

Overall, in EDs there is the need to apply the biopsychosocial model, in multimodal treatments [151], as well as in the sequential management of patients [147, 164], with the cooperation of all the health professionals involved in an active and daily liaison. In EDs, the lack of adequate communication within the treatment staff and an inauthentic care of the somatic, intrapsychic, and relational (family) suffering may collude with the split elements of the patient's self and make treatment iatrogenic and paradoxical.

EDs are still evolving because they represent a modulate and culturally induced way of expressing and, though perversely, alleviating a deep psychosomatic pathology of the development of the self. Moreover, EDs are characterized by complex family and somatopsychic interactions that worsen the organic vulnerability.

Some of the difficulties that emerge in the treatment of patients with EDs are related to the relational style, which is full of indirect anger. A paradoxical request of acceptance and esteem often underlies this relation style, leading to perverted effects. The subtle but stubborn and destructive aggressiveness that causes and maintains these disorders can be directed also against the therapeutic project and sometimes succeeds in nullifying it.

The DCPR proposed are a useful and stimulating tool. In the treatment of EDs, the psychosomatic diagnoses allow a further deepening of diagnosis and a greater attention to the uneasiness and the psychological mechanisms underlying the disorder. A global intervention includes the use of psychotropic drugs for the symptom-related issues (demoralization and irritable mood). Psychotherapy is focused on the identification and expression of emotions, particularly anger. The strengthening of character with expressive psychodynamic psychotherapy may also improve the psychosomatic cores of the ED.

Further studies will address these issues in larger samples, using multivariate statistical analyses. These studies may investigate the use of DCPR to define ad personam the objectives and clinical project and to plan and recalibrate the sequential treatment project and the therapeutic and rehabilitative strategies. Lastly, the DCPR may be useful for the study of outcome predictors of different treatment interventions. Given the promising results of the first use of the DCPR, further research is needed on larger samples to support and validate the role of adjunctive psychosomatic diagnoses in AN, BN, and BED.

Acknowledgements

The authors thank Dr. Carla Gramaglia for her collaboration and helpful suggestions. This work was supported by a grant from Compagnia di San Paolo (512 IT/FA 20003.1888, 10.02.04).

References

1 Van Son GE, van Hoeken D, Bartelds AI, van Furth EF, Hoek HW: Time trends in the incidence of eating disorders: a primary care study in The Netherlands. Int J Eat Disord 2006;39:565–569.
2 Fairburn CG, Harrison PJ: Eating disorders. Lancet 2003;361:407–416.
3 Fairburn CG, Bohn K: Eating disorder NOS (EDNOS): an example of the troublesome 'not otherwise specified' (NOS) category in DSM-IV. Behav Res Ther 2005;43:691–701.
4 Simon J, Schmidt U, Pilling S: The health service use and cost of eating disorders. Psychol Med 2005;35:1543–1551, Review.
5 Striegel-Moore RH, Leslie D, Petrill SA, Garvin V, Rosenheck RA: One-year use and cost of inpatient and outpatient services among female and male patients with eating disorder: evidence from a national database of health insurance claims. Int J Eat Disord 2000;27:381–389.
6 Vandereycken W: The place of inpatient care in the treatment of anorexia nervosa: questions to be answered. Int J Eat Disord 2003;34:409–422.
7 Wyatt SB, Winters KP, Dubbert PM: Overweight and obesity: prevalence, consequences, and causes of a growing public health problem. Am J Med Sci 2006;331:166–174, Review.
8 Garner DM, Garfinkel PE (eds): Handbook of Psychotherapy for Anorexia Nervosa and Bulimia. New York, Guilford Press,1985.
9 Ey H, Bernard P, Brisset CH: Manuel de psychiatrie. Paris, Masson, 1960.

10 Haynal A, Pasini W (1978): Medicina psicosomatica. Milano, Masson, 1979.
11 Adler A: Der Sinn des Lebens. Frankfurt a.M. 1933.
12 Lanfranco F, Gianotti L, Destefanis S, Arvat E, Ghigo E, Camanni F: Endocrine abnormalities in anorexia nervosa. Minerva Endocrinol 2003;28:168–180, Review.
13 Goodyer IM, Park RJ, Netherton CM, Herbert J: Possible role of cortisol and dehydroepiandrosterone in human development and psychopathology. Br J Psychiatry 2001;179:243–249, Review.
14 Keys A, Brozek J, Henschel A, Mickelsen O, Taylor H: The Biology of Human Starvation. Minneapolis, University of Minnesota Press, 1950.
15 Fassino S, Daga GA, Mondelli V, Piero A, Broglio F, Picu A, Giordano R, Baldi M, Arvat E, Ghigo E, Gianotti L: Hormonal and metabolic responses to acute ghrelin administration in patients with bulimia nervosa. Psychoneuroendocrinology 2005;30:534–540.
16 van der Lely AJ, Tschop M, Heiman ML, Ghigo E: Biological, physiological, pathophysiological, and pharmacological aspects of ghrelin. Endocr Rev 2004;25:426–457.
17 Bruch H: Eating Disorders: Obesity, Anorexia Nervosa, and the Person within. New York, Basic Books, 1973.
18 Garfinkel PE, Garner DM, Kaplan AS, Rodin G, Kennedy S: Differential diagnosis of emotional disorders that cause weight loss. Can Med Assoc J 1983;129:939–945.
19 Eisler I, Dare C, Hodes M, Russell G, Dodge E, Le Grange D: Family therapy for adolescent anorexia nervosa: the results of a controlled comparison of two family interventions. J Child Psychol Psychiatry 2000;41:727–736.
20 Le Grange D: The Maudsley family-based treatment for adolescent anorexia nervosa. World Psychiatry 2005;4:142–146.
21 Fassino S, Svrakic D, Abbate-Daga G, Leombruni P, Amianto F, Stanic S, Rovera GG: Anorectic family dynamics: temperament and character data. Compr Psychiatry 2002;43:114–120.
22 Fassino S, Amianto F, Daga GA, Leombruni P, Garzaro L, Levi M, Rovera GG: Bulimic family dynamics: role of parents' personality: a controlled study with the Temperament and Character Inventory. Compr Psychiatry 2003;44:70–77.
23 Minuchin S, Rosman BL, Baker I: Psychosomatic Families: Anorexia Nervosa in Context. Boston, Harvard University Press, 1978.
24 Fava GA, Freyberger HJ, Bech P, Christodoulou G, Sensky T, Theorell T, Wise TN: Diagnostic criteria for use in psychosomatic research. Psychother Psychosom 1995;63:1–8.
25 Jacobi C, Hayward C, de Zwaan M, Kraemer HC, Agras WS: Coming to terms with risk factors for eating disorders: application of risk terminology and suggestions for a general taxonomy. Psychol Bull 2004;130:19–65.
26 Favaro A, Tenconi E, Santonastaso P: Perinatal factors and the risk of developing anorexia nervosa and bulimia nervosa. Arch Gen Psychiatry 2006;63:82–88.
27 Cnattingius S, Hultman CM, Dahl M, Sparen P: Very preterm birth, birth trauma, and the risk of anorexia nervosa among girls. Arch Gen Psychiatry 1999;56:634–638.
28 Penas-Lledo EM, Rodriguez Santos L, Vaz Leal FJ, Waller G: Pattern of birth in restrictive and bulimic eating disorders. Eat Behav 2003;3:325–328.
29 Faravelli C, Giugni A, Salvatori S, Ricca V: Psychopathology after rape. Am J Psychiatry 2004;161:1483–1485.
30 Stice E: Risk and maintenance factors for eating pathology: a meta-analytic review. Psychol Bull 2002;128:825–848.
31 Margo JL: Anorexia nervosa in adolescents. Br J Med Psychol 1985;58(pt 2):193–195.
32 Horesh N, Apter A, Lepkifker E, Ratzoni G, Weizmann R, Tyano S: Life events and severe anorexia nervosa in adolescence. Acta Psychiatr Scand 1995;91:5–9.
33 Schmidt U, Tiller J, Blanchard M, Andrews B, Treasure J: Is there a specific trauma precipitating anorexia nervosa? Psychol Med 1997;27:523–530.
34 Raffi AR, Rondini M, Grandi S, Fava GA: Life events and prodromal symptoms in bulimia nervosa. Psychol Med 2000;30:727–731.
35 Pike KM, Wilfley D, Hilbert A, Fairburn CG, Dohm FA, Striegel-Moore RH: Antecedent life events of binge-eating disorder. Psychiatry Res 2006;142:19–29.
36 Milos GF, Spindler AM, Buddeberg C, Crameri A: Axes I and II comorbidity and treatment experiences in eating disorder subjects. Psychother Psychosom 2003;72:276–285.

37 Grilo CM: Recent research of relationships among eating disorders and personality disorders. Curr Psychiatry Rep 2002;4:18–24, Review.
38 McElroy SL, Kotwal R, Malhotra S, Nelson EB, Keck PE, Nemeroff CB: Are mood disorders and obesity related? A review for the mental health professional. J Clin Psychiatry 2004;65:634–651, quiz 730, Review.
39 Mitchell JE, Mussell MP: Comorbidity and binge eating disorder. Addict Behav 1995;20: 725–732, Review.
40 Striegel-Moore RH, Franko DL: Epidemiology of binge eating disorder. Int J Eat Disord 2003;34 (suppl):S19–S29, Review.
41 O'Brien KM, Vincent NK: Psychiatric comorbidity in anorexia and bulimia nervosa: nature, prevalence, and causal relationships. Clin Psychol Rev 2003;23:57–74, Review.
42 Woodside BD, Staab R: Management of psychiatric comorbidity in anorexia nervosa and bulimia nervosa. CNS Drugs 2006;20:655–663, Review.
43 Porcelli P, De Carne M, Fava GA: Assessing somatization in functional gastrointestinal disorders: integration of different criteria. Psychother Psychosom 2000;69:198–204.
44 Fava GA, Mangelli L, Ruini C: Assessment of psychological distress in the setting of medical disease. Psychother Psychosom 2001;70:171–175.
45 Grandi S, Fabbri S, Tossani E, Mangelli L, Branzi A, Magelli C: Psychological evaluation after cardiac transplantation: the integration of different criteria. Psychother Psychosom 2001;70: 176–183.
46 Rafanelli C, Roncuzzi R, Finos L, Tossani E, Tomba E, Mangelli L, Urbinati S, Pinelli G, Fava GA: Psychological assessment in cardiac rehabilitation. Psychother Psychosom 2003;72: 343–349.
47 Sonino N, Navarrini C, Ruini C, Ottolini F, Paoletta A, Fallo F, Boscaro M, Fava GA: Persistent psychological distress in patients treated for endocrine disease. Psychother Psychosom 2004;73:78–83.
48 Galeazzi GM, Ferrari S, Mackinnon A, Rigatelli M: Interrater reliability, prevalence, and relation to ICD-10 diagnoses of the Diagnostic Criteria for Psychosomatic Research in consultation-liaison psychiatry patients. Psychosomatics 2004;45:386–393.
49 Grassi L, Sabato S, Rossi E, Biancosino B, Marmai L: Use of the diagnostic criteria for psychosomatic research in oncology. Psychother Psychosom 2005;74:100–107.
50 Rafanelli C, Roncuzzi R, Milaneschi Y, Tomba E, Colistro MC, Pancaldi LG, Di Pasquale G: Stressful life events. depression and demoralization as risk factors for acute coronary heart disease. Psychother Psychosom 2005;74:179–184.
51 Ottolini F, Modena MG, Rigatelli M: Prodromal symptoms in myocardial infarction. Psychother Psychosom 2005;74:323–327.
52 Picardi A, Porcelli P, Pasquini P, Fassone G, Mazzotti E, Lega I, Ramieri L, Sagoni E, Abeni D, Tiago A, Fava GA: Integration of multiple criteria for psychosomatic assessment of dermatological patients. Psychosomatics 2006;47:122–128.
53 Mangelli L, Semprini F, Sirri L, Fava GA, Sonino N: Use of the Diagnostic Criteria for Psychosomatic Research (DCPR) in a community sample. Psychosomatics 2006;47:143–146.
54 Cloninger CR, Przybeck TR, Svrakic DM: Temperament and Character Inventory (TCI): A Guide to Its Development and Use. St. Louis, MO, Center for Psychobiology of Personality, Washington University, 1994.
55 Garner DM: Eating Disorder Inventory – 2 professional manual. Odessa, FL, Psychological Assessment Resources, 1991.
56 Spielberger CD: State-Trait Anger Expression Inventory, Research Edition, Professional Manual. Odessa, FL, Psychological Assessment Resources, 1988.
57 Beck AT, Ward CH, Mendelson M, Mock J, Erbaugh J: An inventory for measuring depression. Arch Gen Psychiatry 1961;4:561–571.
58 Troop NA, Schmidt UH, Treasure JL: Feelings and fantasy in eating disorders: a factor analysis of the Toronto Alexithymia Scale. Int J Eat Disord 1995;18:151–157.
59 Rastam M, Gillberg C, Gillberg IC, Johansson M: Alexithymia in anorexia nervosa: a controlled study using the 20-item Toronto Alexithymia Scale. Acta Psychiatr Scand 1997;95:385–388.

60 Sexton MC, Sunday SR, Hurt S, Halmi KA: The relationship between alexithymia, depression, and axis II psychopathology in eating disorder inpatients. Int J Eat Disord 1998;23:277–286.
61 Corcos M, Guilbaud O, Speranza M, Paterniti S, Loas G, Stephan P, Jeammet P: Alexithymia and depression in eating disorders. Psychiatry Res 2000;93:263–266.
62 Zonnevylle-Bender MJ, van Goozen SH, Cohen-Kettenis PT, van Elburg TA, van Engeland H: Emotional functioning in adolescent anorexia nervosa patients – a controlled study. Eur Child Adolesc Psychiatry 2004;13:28–34.
63 Speranza M, Corcos M, Loas G, Stephan P, Guilbaud O, Perez-Diaz F, Venisse JL, Bizouard P, Halfon O, Flament M, Jeammet P: Depressive personality dimensions and alexithymia in eating disorders. Psychiatry Res 2005;135:153–163.
64 Bydlowski S, Corcos M, Jeammet P, Paterniti S, Berthoz S, Laurier C, Chambry J, Consoli SM: Emotion-processing deficits in eating disorders. Int J Eat Disord 2005;37:321–329.
65 Iancu I, Cohen E, Yehuda YB, Kotler M: Treatment of eating disorders improves eating symptoms but not alexithymia and dissociation proneness. Compr Psychiatry 2006;47:189–193.
66 Kessler H, Schwarze M, Filipic S, Traue HC, von Wietersheim J: Alexithymia and facial emotion recognition in patients with eating disorders. Int J Eat Disord 2006;39:245–251.
67 Fassino S, Leombruni P, Piero A, Daga GA, Amianto F, Rovera G, Rovera GG: Temperament and character in obese women with and without binge eating disorder. Compr Psychiatry 2002;43: 431–437.
68 Gilboa-Schechtman E, Avnon L, Zubery E, Jeczmien P: Emotional processing in eating disorders: specific impairment or general distress related deficiency? Depress Anxiety 2006;23:331–339.
69 Fassino S, Abbate-Daga G, Amianto F, Leombruni P, Boggio S, Rovera GG: Temperament and character profile of eating disorders: a controlled study with the Temperament and Character Inventory. Int J Eat Disord 2002;32:412–425.
70 Picardi A, Toni A, Caroppo E: Stability of alexithymia and its relationships with the 'big five' factors, temperament, character, and attachment style. Psychother Psychosom 2005;74:371–378.
71 Grabe HJ, Spitzer C, Freyberger HJ: Alexithymia and the temperament and character model of personality. Psychother Psychosom 2001;70:261–267.
72 Bruch H: Obesity and anorexia nervosa. Psychosomatics 1978;19:208–212.
73 Canetti L, Bachar E, Berry EM: Food and emotion. Behav Processes 2002;60:157–164.
74 Fava GA, Sonino N: Psychosomatic medicine: emerging trends and perspectives. Psychother Psychosom 2000;69:184–197.
75 Truglia E, Mannucci E, Lassi S, Rotella CM, Faravelli C, Ricca V: Aggressiveness, anger and eating disorders: a review. Psychopathology 2006;39:55–68.
76 Hinrichsen H, Wright F, Waller G, Meyer C: Social anxiety and coping strategies in the eating disorders. Eat Behav 2003;4:117–126.
77 Edman JL, Yates A, Aruguete MS, DeBord KA: Negative emotion and disordered eating among obese college students. Eat Behav 2005;6:308–317, Epub 2005 Jun 13.
78 Fassino S, Leombruni P, Piero A, Abbate-Daga G, Giacomo Rovera G: Mood, eating attitudes, and anger in obese women with and without Binge Eating Disorder. J Psychosom Res 2003;54:559–566.
79 Masheb RM, Grilo CM: Emotional overeating and its associations with eating disorder psychopathology among overweight patients with binge eating disorder. Int J Eat Disord 2006;39: 141–146.
80 Welldon A: Mother, Madonna, Whore. New York, Guilford, 1988.
81 Lane A: Relationships between attitudes towards eating disorders and mood. J Sci Med Sport 2003;6:144–154.
82 Fichter MM, Quadflieg N, Rief W: Course of multi-impulsive bulimia. Psychol Med 1994;24: 591–604.
83 Tiller J, Schmidt U, Ali S, Treasure J: Patterns of punitiveness in women with eating disorders. Int J Eat Disord 1995;17:365–371.
84 Youssef G, Plancherel B, Laget J, Corcos M, Flament MF, Halfon O: Personality trait risk factors for attempted suicide among young women with eating disorders. Eur Psychiatry 2004;19: 131–139.
85 Abbate-Daga G, Piero A, Gramaglia C, Fassino S: Factors related to severity of vomiting behaviors in bulimia nervosa. Psychiatry Res 2005;134:75–84.

86 Tozzi F, Thornton LM, Mitchell J, Fichter MM, Klump KL, Lilenfeld LR, Reba L, Strober M, Kaye WH, Bulik CM: Price Foundation Collaborative Group. Features associated with laxative abuse in individuals with eating disorders. Psychosom Med 2006;68:470–477.
87 Johnson C, Maddi KL: The etiology of bulimia: biopsychosocial perspectives. Adolesc Psychiatry 1986;13:253–273.
88 Meyer C, Leung N, Waller G, Perkins S, Paice N, Mitchell J: Anger and bulimic psychopathology: gender differences in a nonclinical group. Int J Eat Disord 2005;37:69–71.
89 Fassino S, Daga GA, Piero A, Leombruni P, Rovera GG: Anger and personality in eating disorders. J Psychosom Res 2001;51:757–764.
90 Shugar G, Krueger S: Aggressive family communication, weight gain, and improved eating attitudes during systemic family therapy for anorexia nervosa. Int J Eat Disord 1995;17:23–31.
91 Steiger H, Goldstein C, Mongrain M, Van Der Feen M: Description of eating disorders, psychiatric and normal women along cognitive and psychodynamic dimensions. Int J Eat Disord 1990;9:129–140.
92 Strober M, Humphrey LL: Familial contributions to the etiology and course of anorexia nervosa and bulimia. J Consult Clin Psychol 1987;55:654–659.
93 Fahy TA, Eisler I, Russell GF: Personality disorder and treatment response in bulimia nervosa. Br J Psychiatry 1993;162:765–770.
94 Jimerson DC, Lesem MD, Hegg AP, Brewerton TD: Serotonin in human eating disorders. Ann N Y Acad Sci 1990;600:532–544.
95 Brewerton TD, Jimerson DC: Studies of serotonin function in anorexia nervosa. Psychiatry Res 1996;62:31–42.
96 Fava M, Rappe SM, West J, Herzog DB: Anger attacks in eating disorders. Psychiatry Res 1995;56:205–212.
97 Fassino S, Abbate-Daga G, Amianto F, Leombruni P, Fornas B, Garzaro L, D'Ambrosio G, Rovera GG: Outcome predictors in anorectic patients after 6 months of multimodal treatment. Psychother Psychosom 2001;70:201–208.
98 Cloninger CR: A practical way to diagnosis personality disorder: a proposal. J Personal Disord 2000;14:99–108.
99 American Psychiatric Association: Practice guideline for the treatment of patients with eating disorders (Revision). Am J Psychiatry 2000;157:1–39.
100 American Psychiatric Association: Practice Guideline for the Treatment of Patients with Eating Disorders, ed 3. Am J Psychiatry 2006;163(suppl):7.
101 Fassino S, Daga GA, Piero A, Rovera GG: Dropout from brief psychotherapy in anorexia nervosa. Psychother Psychosom 2002;71:200–206.
102 Grilo GM, Masheb RM, Wilson GT: A comparison of different methods for assessing the features of eating disorders in patients with binge eating disorder. J Consult Clin Psychol 2001;69:317.
103 Mangelli L, Fava GA, Grandi S, Grassi L, Ottolini F, Porcelli P, Rafanelli C, Rigatelli M, Sonino N: Assessing demoralization and depression in the setting of medical disease. J Clin Psychiatry 2005;66:391–394.
104 Fava GA, Ruini C, Rafanelli C: Psychometric theory is an obstacle to the progress of clinical research. Psychother Psychosom 2004;73:145–148.
105 Fassino S, Abbate-Daga G, Pierò A: Il trattamento dei disturbi del comportamento alimentare secondo la prospettiva della psicologia individuale. Riv Psicologia Individuale 2004;56:16–34.
106 Zonnevylle-Bender MJ, van Goozen SH, Cohen-Kettenis PT, van Elburg A, de Wildt M, Stevelmans E, van Engeland H: Emotional functioning in anorexia nervosa patients: adolescents compared to adults. Depress Anxiety 2004;19:35–42.
107 Montebarocci O, Codispoti M, Surcinelli P, Franzoni E, Baldaro B, Rossi N: Alexithymia in female patients with eating disorders. Eat Weight Disord 2006;11:14–21.
108 Fukunishi I, Koyama K: Relations of alexithymic characteristics with eating attitudes and hostility in female college students. Psychol Rep 2001;88(pt 2):1245–1250.
109 Fassino S, Abbate-Daga G, Leombruni P, Amianto F, Rovera G, Rovera GG: Temperament and character in Italian men with anorexia nervosa: a controlled study with the temperament and character inventory. J Nerv Ment Dis 2001;189:788–794.
110 Lee M, Shafran R: Information processing biases in eating disorders. Clin Psychol Rev 2004;24:215–238.

111 Zonnevylle-Bender MJ, van Goozen SH, Cohen-Kettenis PT, Jansen LM, van Elburg A, Engeland H: Adolescent anorexia nervosa patients have a discrepancy between neurophysiological responses and self-reported emotional arousal to psychosocial stress. Psychiatry Res 2005;135:45–52.
112 Fassino S, Piero A, Daga GA, Leombruni P, Mortara P, Rovera GG: Attentional biases and frontal functioning in anorexia nervosa. Int J Eat Disord 2002;31:274–283.
113 Espina A: Alexithymia in parents of daughters with eating disorders: its relationships with psychopathological and personality variables. J Psychosom Res 2003;55:553–560.
114 De Panfilis C, Rabbaglio P, Rossi C, Zita G, Maggini C: Body image disturbance, parental bonding and alexithymia in patients with eating disorders. Psychopathology 2003;36:239–246.
115 Legorreta G, Bull RH, Kiely MC: Alexithymia and symbolic function in the obese. Psychother Psychosom 1988;50:88–94.
116 Clerici M, Albonetti S, Papa R, Penati G, Invernizzi G: Alexithymia and obesity. Study of the impaired symbolic function by the Rorschach test. Psychother Psychosom 1992;57:88–93.
117 de Zwaan M, Bach M, Mitchell JE, Ackard D, Specker SM, Pyle RL, Pakesch G: Alexithymia, obesity, and binge eating disorder. Int J Eat Disord 1995;17:135–140.
118 Morosin A, Riva G: Alexithymia in a clinical sample of obese women. Psychol Rep 1997;80: 387–394.
119 Pinaquy S, Chabrol H, Simon C, Louvet JP, Barbe P: Emotional eating, alexithymia, and binge-eating disorder in obese women. Obes Res 2003;11:195–201.
120 Wheeler K, Greiner P, Boulton M: Exploring alexithymia, depression, and binge eating in self-reported eating disorders in women. Perspect Psychiatr Care 2005;41:114–123.
121 Carano A, De Berardis D, Gambi F, Di Paolo C, Campanella D, Pelusi L, Sepede G, Mancini E, La Rovere R, Salini G, Cotellessa C, Salerno RM, Ferro FM: Alexithymia and body image in adult outpatients with binge eating disorder. Int J Eat Disord 2006;39:332–340.
122 Bankier B, Littman AB: Psychiatric disorders and coronary heart disease in women – a still neglected topic: review of the literature from 1971 to 2000. Psychother Psychosom 2002;71:133–140.
123 Larson JA: New perspectives on type A behavior: a psychiatric point of view. Int J Psychiatry Med 1993;23:179–194.
124 Bulik CM, Tozzi F, Anderson C, Mazzeo SE, Aggen S, Sullivan PF: The relation between eating disorders and components of perfectionism. Am J Psychiatry 2003;160:366–368.
125 Brunner RL, Maloney MJ, Daniels S, Mays W, Farrell M: A controlled study of type A behavior and psychophysiologic responses to stress in anorexia nervosa. Psychiatry Res 1989;30:223–230.
126 Sifneos PE: The prevalence of 'alexithymic' characteristics in psychosomatic patients. Psychother Psychosom 1973;22:255–262.
127 Wise TN, Mann LS, Randell P: The stability of alexithymia in depressed patients. Psychopathology 1995;28:173.
128 Podar I, Hannus A, Allik J: Personality and affectivity characteristics associated with eating disorders: a comparison of eating disordered, weight-preoccupied, and normal samples. J Pers Assess 1999;73:133–147.
129 Rosenvinge JH, Martinussen M, Ostensen E: The comorbidity of eating disorders and personality disorders: a meta-analytic review of studies published between 1983 and 1998. Eat Weight Disord 2000;5:52–61.
130 Halmi KA, Garfinkel PE: Eating disorders; in Gabbard GO, Atkinson SD (eds): Synopsis of Treatments of Psychiatric Disorders, ed 2. American Psychiatric Association, 1996.
131 Herzog DB, Keller MB, Lavori PW, Kenny GM, Sacks NR: The prevalence of personality disorders in 210 women with eating disorders. J Clin Psychiatry 1992;53:147–152.
132 Wonderlich SA, Fullerton D, Swift WJ, Klein MH: Five-year outcome from eating disorders: relevance of personality disorders. Int J Eat Disord 1994;15:233–243.
133 Matsunaga H, Kaye WH, McConaha C, Plotnicov K, Pollice C, Rao R: Personality disorders among subjects recovered from eating disorders. Int J Eat Disord 2000;27:353–357.
134 Cloninger CR: A systematic method for clinical description and classification of personality variants. A proposal. Arch Gen Psychiatry 1987;44:573–588.
135 Svrakic DM, Whitehead C, Przybeck TR, Cloninger CR: Differential diagnosis of personality disorders by the seven-factor model of temperament and character. Arch Gen Psychiatry 1993;50: 991–999.

136 Peirson AR, Heuchert JW, Thomala L, Berk M, Plein H, Cloninger CR: Relationship between serotonin and the temperament and character inventory. Psychiatry Res 1999;89:29–37.
137 Gendall KA, Joyce PR, Sullivan PF, Bulik CM: Personality and dimensions of dietary restraint. Int J Eat Disord 1998;24:371–379.
138 Brewerton TD, Dorn LJ, Bishop ER: The Tridimensional Personality Questionnaire in eating disorders. Biol Psychiatry 1992;31:91A.
139 Brewerton TD, Hand LD, Bishop ER Jr: The Tridimensional Personality Questionnaire in eating disorder patients. Int J Eat Disord 1993;14:213–218.
140 Strober M: Disorders of the self in anorexia nervosa: an organismic-developmental perspective; in Johnson C (ed): Psychodynamic Theory and Treatment of Anorexia Nervosa and Bulimia. New York: Guilford Publishers, 1992, pp 354–373.
141 Casper RC, Hedeker D, McClough JF: Personality dimensions in eating disorders and their relevance for subtyping. J Am Acad Child Adolesc Psychiatry 1992;31:830–840.
142 Bulik CM, Sullivan PF, Weltzin TE, Kaye WH: Temperament in eating disorders. Int J Eat Disord 1995;17:251–261.
143 Klump KL, Bulik CM, Pollice C, Halmi KA, Fichter MM, Berrettini WH, Devlin B, Strober M, Kaplan A, Woodside DB, Treasure J, Shabbout M, Lilenfeld LR, Plotnicov KH, Kaye WH: Temperament and character in women with anorexia nervosa. J Nerv Ment Dis 2000;188: 559–567.
144 Diaz-Marsa M, Carrasco JL, Saiz J: A study of temperament and personality in anorexia and bulimia nervosa. J Personal Disord 2000;14:352–359.
145 Mitszushima H, Ono Y, Asai M: TCI Temperamental scores in bulimia nervosa patients and normal women with and without diet experiences. Acta Psychiatr Scand 1998;98:228–230.
146 Diaz Marsa M, Carrasco Perera JL, Prieto Lopez R, Saiz Ruiz J: The role of the personality in the feeding behavior disorders. Actas Esp Psiquiatr 1999;27:43–50.
147 Fassino S, Piero A, Levi M, Gramaglia C, Amianto F, Leombruni P, Abbate-Daga G: Psychological treatment of eating disorders. A review of the literature. Panminerva Med 2004;46:189–198.
148 Gundel H, Lopez-Sala A, Ceballos-Baumann AO, Deus J, Cardoner N, Marten-Mittag B, Soriano-Mas C, Pujol J: Alexithymia correlates with the size of the right anterior cingulate. Psychosom Med 2004;66:132–140.
149 Evren C, Evren B: The relationship of suicide attempt history with childhood abuse and neglect. alexithymia and temperament and character dimensions of personality in substance dependents. Nord J Psychiatry 2006;60:263–269.
150 Evren C, Evren B: Self-mutilation in substance-dependent patients and relationship with childhood abuse and neglect, alexithymia and temperament and character dimensions of personality. Drug Alcohol Depend 2005;80:15–22.
151 Halmi KA: The multimodal treatment of eating disorders. World Psychiatry 2005;4:69–73.
152 Fassino S, Amianto F, Gramaglia C, Facchini F, Abbate-Daga G: Temperament and character in eating disorders: ten years of studies. Eat Weight Disord 2004;9:81–90.
153 Beales DL, Dolton R: Eating disordered patients: personality, alexithymia, and implications for primary care. Br J Gen Pract 2000;50:21–26.
154 De Groot JM, Rodin G, Olmsted MP: Alexithymia, depression, and treatment outcome in bulimia nervosa. Compr Psychiatry 1995;36:53–60.
155 Fassino S, Piero A, Gramaglia C, Abbate-Daga G: Clinical, psychopathological and personality correlates of interoceptive awareness in anorexia nervosa, bulimia nervosa and obesity. Psychopathology 2004;37:168–174.
156 Gabbard GO: Psychodynamic Psychiatry in Clinical Practice. The DSM – IV Edition. Washington DC, American Psychiatric Press, 1994.
157 Dare C, Eisler I, Russell G, Treasure J, Dodge L: Psychological therapies for adults with anorexia nervosa: randomised controlled trial of out-patient treatments. Br J Psychiatry 2001;178:216–221.
158 Hay PJ, Bacaltchuk J, Stefano S: Psychotherapy for bulimia nervosa and binging. Cochrane Database Syst Rev 2004;CD000562, Review.
159 Agras WS, Walsh T, Fairburn CG, Wilson GT, Kraemer HC: A multicenter comparison of cognitive-behavioral therapy and interpersonal psychotherapy for bulimia nervosa. Arch Gen Psychiatry 2000;57:459–466.

160 Vaidya V: Cognitive behavior therapy of binge eating disorder; in Vaidya V (ed): Health and Treatment Strategies in Obesity. Adv Psychosom Med. Basel, Karger, 2006, vol 27, pp 86–93.
161 Fairburn CG: Evidence-base treatment of anorexia nervosa. Int J Eat Disord 2005;37:S26–S30.
162 Garner DM, Garfinkel PE: Handbook of Treatment for Eating Disorders, ed 2. New York, Guilford Press, 1997.
163 Dalle Grave R, Ricca V, Todesco T: The stepped-care approach in anorexia nervosa and bulimia nervosa: progress and problems. Eat Weight Disord 2001;6:81–89.
164 Fava GA: Sequential treatment: a new way of integrating pharmacotherapy and psychotherapy. Psychother Psychosom 1999;68:227–229.
165 Svrakic DM, Cloninger R, Stanic S, Fassino S: Classification of personality disorders: implications for treatment and research; in Soares JC, Gershon S (eds): Handbook of Medical Psychiatry. New York, Marcel Dekker, 2003, pp 117–148.
166 Kaplan AS, Garfinkel PE: Difficulties in treating patients with eating disorders: a review of patient and clinician variables. Can J Psychiatry 1999;44:665–670.
167 Peggy CP: The Secret Language of Eating Disorders. Random House Value Pub, 1997.
168 Godart N, Atger F, Perdereau F, Agman G, Rein Z, Corcos M, Jeammet P: Treatment of adolescent patients with eating disorders: description of a psychodynamic approach in clinical practice. Eat Weight Disord 2004;9:224–227.
169 Bruch H: Treatment in anorexia nervosa. Int J Psychoanal Psychother 1982–1983;9:303–312.
170 Gabbard GO, Atkinson S: Synopsis of Treatment of Psychiatric Disorder, ed 2. Washington, American Psychiatric Press.
171 Russell GFM: Anorexia nervosa and bulimia nervosa; in Russell GFM, Hersov L (a cura di): Handbook of Psychiatry. Cambridge, United Kingdom, Cambridge University Press, 1983, pp 1047–1056.
172 Hudson J, Rapee R (eds): Psychopathology and the Family. Amsterdam, Elsevier, 2005.
173 Fassino S, Svrakic D, Abbate-Daga G, Leombruni P, Amianto F, Stanic S, Rovera GG: Anorectic family dynamics: temperament and character data. Compr Psychiatry 2002;43:114–120.
174 Eisler I, Dare C, Russell GF, Szmukler G, le Grange D, Dodge E: Family and individual therapy in anorexia nervosa. A 5-year follow-up. Arch Gen Psychiatry 1997;54:1025–1030.
175 Lock J, Agras WS, Bryson S, Kraemer HC: A comparison of short- and long-term family therapy for adolescent anorexia nervosa. J Am Acad Child Adolesc Psychiatry 2005;44:632–639.
176 McIntosh VV, Jordan J, Carter FA, Luty SE, McKenzie JM, Bulik CM, Frampton CM, Joyce PR: Three psychotherapies for anorexia nervosa: a randomized controlled trial. Am J Psychiatry 2005;162:741–747.
177 Eisler I, Dare C, Hodes M, Russell G, Dodge E, Le Grange D: Family therapy for adolescent anorexia nervosa: the results of a controlled comparison of two family interventions. J Child Psychol Psychiatry 2000;41:727–736.
178 Keen DR: Anorexia nervosa: an adlerian perspective on etiology and treatment. Individ Psychol 1996;52:386–405.
179 Frank H, Paris J: Recollections of family experience in borderline patients. Arch Gen Psychiatry 1981;38:1031–1034.
180 Corey G: Adlerian therapy; in Corey G (a cura di): Theory and Practice of Counselling and Psychotherapy. Pacific Grove, CA, Brooks/Cole, 1996, pp 53–70.
181 McCormick D, Kottman T, Ashby J: Conceptualization and treatment of the bulimic client from an adlerian perspective. Individ Psychol 1996;52:406–419.
182 Sperry L, Carlson J: Psychopathology and Psychotherapy: From DSM IV Diagnosis to Treatment. Washington DC, Accelerated Development, 1996.

Prof. Secondo Fassino
Università degli Studi di Torino, Department of Neuroscience, Psychiatric Institute
Via Cherasco, 11
IT–10126 Torino (Italy)
Tel. +39 011 6634 848, Fax +39 011 673 473, E-Mail secondo.fassino@unito.it

Porcelli P, Sonino N (eds): Psychological Factors Affecting Medical Conditions. A New Classification for DSM-V. Adv Psychosom Med. Basel, Karger, 2007, vol 28, pp 169–173

Appendix 1. Diagnostic Criteria for Psychosomatic Research

Fava GA, Freyberger HJ, Bech P, Christodoulou G, Sensky T, Theorell T, Wise TN: Diagnostic criteria for use in psychosomatic research. Psychother Psychosom 1995;63:1–8.

Health Anxiety (A through B are required)

A A generic worry about illness, concern about pain and bodily preoccupations (tendency to amplify somatic sensations) of less than 6 months' duration

B Worries and fears readily respond to appropriate medical reassurance, even though new worries may ensue after some time

Thanatophobia (A through C are required)

A Attacks with the sense of impending death and/or conviction of dying soon, even though there is no objective medical reason for such fear

B Marked and persistent fear and avoidance of news which reminds of death (e.g. funerals, obituary notices); exposure to these stimulus almost invariably provokes an immediate anxiety response

C The avoidance, anxious anticipation and distress interfere significantly with the person's level of functioning

Disease Phobia (A through C are required)

A Persistent, unfounded fear of suffering from a specific disease (e.g. AIDS, cancer), with doubts remaining despite adequate examination and reassurance
B Fears tend to manifest themselves in attacks rather than in constant, chronic worries as in hypochondriasis; panic attacks may be an associated feature
C The object of fears does not change with time and duration of symptoms exceeds 6 months

Illness Denial (A through B are required)

A Persistent denial of having a physical disorder and of need of treatment (e.g. lack of compliance, delayed seeking of medical attention for serious and persistent symptoms, counterphobic behavior), as a reaction to the symptoms, signs, diagnosis or medical treatment of a physical illness
B The patient has been provided a lucid and accurate appraisal of the medical situation and management to be followed

Persistent Somatization (A through B are required)

A Functional medical disorders (e.g. fibromyalgia, fatigue, esophageal motility disorders, nonulcer dyspepsia, irritable bowel syndrome, neurocirculatory asthenia, urethral syndromes), whose duration exceeds 6 months, causing distress, or repeated medical care, or resulting in impaired quality of life
B Additional symptoms of autonomic arousal involving also other organ systems (e.g. palpitations, sweating, tremor, flushing) and exaggerated side effects from medical therapy are presented, indicating low sensation of pain thresholds and high suggestionability

Conversion Symptoms (A through C are required)

A One or more symptoms or deficits affecting voluntary motor or sensory function, characterized by lack of anatomical of physiological plausibility, and/or absence of expected physical signs or laboratory findings, and/or inconsistent clinical characteristics; if symptoms of autonomic arousal (e.g. palpitations, sweating, tremor, flushing) or functional medical disorder are present (e.g. fibromyalgia, fatigue, esophageal motility disorders, nonulcer dyspepsia, irritable bowel syndrome, neurocirculatory asthenia, urethral syndromes), conversion symptoms should be prominent, causing distress, or repeated medical care, or resulting in impaired quality of life

B At least 2 of the following features are present:
- **1** ambivalence in symptom reporting (e.g. the patient appears relaxed or unconcerned as he/she describes distressing symptoms)
- **2** histrionic personality features (colorful and dramatic expression, language and appearance, demanding dependency, high suggestionability, rapid mood changes)
- **3** precipitation of symptoms by psychological stress, the association of which the patient is unaware
- **4** history of similar physical symptoms experienced by the patient, or observed in someone else, of wished on someone else

C Appropriate medical evaluation uncovers no organic pathology to account for physical complaints

Functional Somatic Symptoms Secondary to a Psychiatric Disorder (A through C are required)

A Symptoms of autonomic arousal (e.g. palpitations, sweating, tremor, flushing) or functional medical disorder (e.g. irritable bowel syndrome, fibromyalgia, neurocirculatory asthenia), causing distress, or repeated medical care, or resulting in impaired quality of life

B Appropriate medical evaluation uncovers no organic pathology to account for the physical complaints

C A psychiatric disorder (which includes the involved somatic symptoms within its manifestations) preceded the onset of functional somatic symptoms (e.g. panic disorder and cardiac symptoms)